Endocrinology

Editors

ANDREW B. MUIR
SUSAN R. ROSE

CLINICS IN PERINATOLOGY

www.perinatology.theclinics.com

Consulting Editor
LUCKY JAIN

March 2018 • Volume 45 • Number 1

ELSEVIER

1600 John F. Kennedy Boulevard ● Suite 1800 ● Philadelphia, Pennsylvania, 19103-2899

http://www.theclinics.com

CLINICS IN PERINATOLOGY Volume 45, Number 1
March 2018 ISSN 0095-5108, ISBN-13: 978-0-323-58168-4

Editor: Kerry Holland
Developmental Editor: Casey Potter

Clinics in Perinatology (ISSN 0095-5108) is published quarterly by Elsevier Inc., 360 Park Avenue South, New York, NY 10010-1710. Months of issue are March, June, September, and December. Business and Editorial Offices: 1600 John F. Kennedy Blvd., Ste. 1800, Philadelphia, PA 19103-2899. Customer Service Office: 3251 Riverport Lane, Maryland Heights, MO 63043. Periodicals postage paid at New York, NY and additional mailing offices. Subscription prices are $299.00 per year (US individuals), $548.00 per year (US institutions), $351.00 per year (Canadian individuals), $670.00 per year (Canadian institutions), $433.00 per year (international individuals), $670.00 per year (international institutions), $100.00 per year (US students), and $195.00 per year (Canadian and international students). International air speed delivery is included in all Clinics subscription prices. All prices are subject to change without notice. **POSTMASTER:** Send address changes to *Clinics in Perinatology*, Elsevier Health Sciences Division, Subscription Customer Service, 3251 Riverport Lane, Maryland Heights, MO 63043. **Customer Service: Telephone: 1-800-654-2452** (U.S. and Canada); **1-314-447-8871** (outside U.S. and Canada). **Fax: 1-314-447-8029.** E-mail: **journalscustomerservice-usa@elsevier.com** (for print support); **journalsonlinesupport-usa@elsevier.com** (for online support).

Reprints. For copies of 100 or more, of articles in this publication, please contact the Commercial Reprints Department, Elsevier Inc., 360 Park Avenue South, New York, NY 10010-1710. Tel. 212-633-3874; Fax: 212-633-3820; E-mail: reprints@elsevier.com.

Clinics in Perinatology is also published in Spanish by McGraw-Hill Interamericana Editores S.A., P.O. Box 5-237, 06500 Mexico D.F., Mexico.

Clinics in Perinatology is covered in *MEDLINE/PubMed (Index Medicus) Current Contents, Excepta Medica, BIOSIS and ISI/BIOMED.*

Contributors

CONSULTING EDITOR

LUCKY JAIN, MD, MBA
Richard W. Blumberg Professor and Chairman, Department of Pediatrics, Emory University School of Medicine, Chief Academic Officer, Children's Healthcare of Atlanta, Atlanta, Georgia, USA

EDITORS

ANDREW B. MUIR, MD
Marcus Professor of Pediatrics, Pediatric Endocrinology, Emory University, Atlanta, Georgia, USA

SUSAN R. ROSE, MD, MEd
Professor Emerita, Pediatrics and Pediatric Endocrinology, Cincinnati Children's Hospital Medical Center, University of Cincinnati College of Medicine, Cincinnati, Ohio, USA

AUTHORS

PHILIPPE F. BACKELJAUW, MD
Professor of Pediatrics, Division of Endocrinology, Cincinnati Children's Hospital Medical Center, University of Cincinnati College of Medicine, Cincinnati, Ohio, USA

ANDREW J. BAUER, MD
Division of Endocrinology and Diabetes, The Children's Hospital of Philadelphia, Director, The Thyroid Center, Philadelphia, Pennsylvania, USA

MONIKA CHAUDHARI, MD
Associate Professor, Department of Pediatrics, Division of Endocrinology, Nationwide Children's Hospital, The Ohio State University, Columbus, Ohio, USA

DIVA D. DE LEÓN, MD, MSCE
Associate Professor, Department of Pediatrics, Division of Endocrinology and Diabetes, The Children's Hospital of Philadelphia, Perelman School of Medicine University of Pennsylvania, Philadelphia, Pennsylvania, USA

SIRI ATMA W. GREELEY, MD, PhD
Assistant Professor of Pediatrics and Medicine, Section of Adult and Pediatric Endocrinology, Diabetes, and Metabolism, Kovler Diabetes Center, The University of Chicago Medicine, Chicago, Illinois, USA

HEIDI E. KARPEN, MD
Assistant Professor of Pediatrics, Emory University School of Medicine, Atlanta, Georgia, USA

MICHELLE BLANCO LEMELMAN, MD
Pediatric Endocrinology Fellow, Section of Adult and Pediatric Endocrinology, Diabetes, and Metabolism, Chicago, Illinois, USA

LISA LETOURNEAU, MPH, RD, LDN
Study Coordinator, Monogenic Diabetes Registry, Kovler Diabetes Center, The University of Chicago Medicine, Chicago, Illinois, USA

KATHERINE LORD, MD
Assistant Professor, Department of Pediatrics, Division of Endocrinology and Diabetes, The Children's Hospital of Philadelphia, The Perelman School of Medicine University of Pennsylvania, Philadelphia, Pennsylvania, USA

SISI M. NAMOC, MD
National Child Health Institute, Breña - Lima, Peru

JOHN S. PARKS, MD, PhD
Professor of Pediatrics, Emeritus, Emory University School of Medicine, Atlanta, Georgia, USA

JACOB M. REDEL, MD
Clinical Fellow, Division of Endocrinology, Cincinnati Children's Hospital Medical Center, University of Cincinnati College of Medicine, Cincinnati, Ohio, USA

SUSAN R. ROSE, MD, MEd
Professor Emerita, Pediatrics and Pediatric Endocrinology, Cincinnati Children's Hospital Medical Center, University of Cincinnati College of Medicine, Cincinnati, Ohio, USA

STEPHANIE L. SAMUELS, MD
Division of Endocrinology and Diabetes, The Children's Hospital of Philadelphia, Philadelphia, Pennsylvania, USA

SUSAN M. SCOTT, MD, JD
Professor Emerita, School of Medicine, The University of New Mexico, Albuquerque, New Mexico, USA

JONATHAN L. SLAUGHTER, MD, MPH
Assistant Professor, Department of Pediatrics, Division of Neonatology, Center for Perinatal Research, Nationwide Children's Hospital, The Ohio State University, Columbus, Ohio, USA

CONSTANTINE A. STRATAKIS, MD, D(Med)Sc
Section on Endocrinology and Genetics, Developmental Endocrine Oncology and Genetics Group, Pediatric Endocrinology Inter-institute Training Program, Eunice Kennedy Shriver National Institute of Child Health and Human Development (NICHD), National Institutes of Health (NIH), NIH-Clinical Research Center, Bethesda, Maryland, USA

CHRISTINA TATSI, MD, PhD
Section on Endocrinology and Genetics, Developmental Endocrine Oncology and Genetics Group, Pediatric Endocrinology Inter-institute Training Program, Eunice Kennedy Shriver National Institute of Child Health and Human Development (NICHD), National Institutes of Health (NIH), NIH-Clinical Research Center, Bethesda, Maryland, USA

ARI J. WASSNER, MD
Director, Thyroid Program, Division of Endocrinology, Boston Children's Hospital, Assistant Professor of Pediatrics, Harvard Medical School, Boston, Massachusetts, USA

Contents

> Congenital hypothyroidism is common and can cause severe neurodevelopmental morbidity. Prompt diagnosis and treatment are critical to optimizing long-term outcomes. Universal newborn screening is an important tool for detecting congenital hypothyroidism, but awareness of its limitations, repeated screening in high-risk infants, and a high index of clinical suspicion are needed to ensure that all affected infants are appropriately identified and treated. Careful evaluation will usually reveal the etiology of congenital hypothyroidism, which may inform treatment and prognosis. Early and adequate treatment with levothyroxine results in excellent neurodevelopmental outcomes for most patients with congenital hypothyroidism.

> Patients in the neonatal intensive care unit (NICU) are at high risk for abnormal thyroid function testing because of illness and preterm birth. Preterm infants are born before hypothalamic-pituitary-thyroid axis maturation, and the normal feedback mechanisms that regulate thyroid hormone production remain immature. Preterm and sick infants may develop hypothyroidism even if routine thyroid screening tests collected in the first several days after birth are normal. This article reviews normal hypothalamic-pituitary-thyroid axis maturation, thyroid hormone testing and interpretation in the NICU, and the current evidence for and against levothyroxine treatment of NICU patients with borderline abnormal thyroid function testing.

> Neonatal thyrotoxicosis (hyperthyroidism) is less prevalent than congenital hypothyroidism; however, it can lead to significant morbidity and mortality if not promptly recognized and adequately treated. Most cases are transient, secondary to maternal autoimmune hyperthyroidism (Graves disease [GD]). This article summarizes recommendations for screening and management of hyperthyroidism in both the fetal and neonatal periods, with a focus on neonatal thyrotoxicosis secondary to maternal GD. Early monitoring and treatment are crucial for optimizing short-term and long-term patient outcomes.

Neonatal Cushing syndrome (CS) is most commonly caused by exogenous administration of glucocorticoids and rarely by endogenous hypercortisolemia. Adrenal lesions are the most common cause of endogenous CS in neonates and infants, and adrenocortical tumors (ACTs) represent most cases. Many ACTs develop in the context of a *TP53* gene mutation, which causes Li-Fraumeni syndrome. More rarely, neonatal CS presents as part of other syndromes such as McCune-Albright syndrome or Beckwith-Wiedemann syndrome. Management usually includes resection of the primary tumor with or without additional medical treatment, but manifestations may persist after resolution of hypercortisolemia.

The perinatal clinician needs to understand certain essential concepts when encountering an infant with a suspected or confirmed diagnosis of Turner syndrome. This article describes the key clinical features that should prompt testing, the appropriate diagnostic workup, the necessary screening required after diagnosis, and how to best approach family counseling.

Most bone formation and mineralization occurs late in gestation. Accretion of adequate minerals is a key element of this process and is often interrupted through preterm birth. In utero, mineral transport is accomplished via active transport across the placenta and does not require fetal hormone input. Postnatal mineral homeostasis requires a balance of actions of parathyroid hormone, calcitonin, and vitamin D on target organs. Preterm birth, asphyxia, acidosis, and prolonged parenteral nutrition increase the risk of mineral imbalance and metabolic bone disease (MBD). Aggressive postnatal nutrition is key to preventing and treating MBD in preterm infants.

PROGRAM OBJECTIVE
The goal of *Clinics in Perinatology* is to keep practicing perinatologists, neonatologists, obstetricians, practicing physicians and residents up to date with current clinical practice in perinatology by providing timely articles reviewing the state of the art in patient care.

TARGET AUDIENCE
Perinatologists, neonatologists, obstetricians, practicing physicians, residents and healthcare professionals who provide patient care utilizing findings from *Clinics in Perinatology*.

LEARNING OBJECTIVES
Upon completion of this activity, participants will be able to:
1. Review Neonatal Cushing Syndrome, congenital hypothyroidism.
2. Discuss neonatal diabetes mellitus, hyperinsulinism, and hypopituitarism.
3. Recognize Turner Syndrome and mineral homeostasis and effects on bone mineralization.

ACCREDITATION
The Elsevier Office of Continuing Medical Education (EOCME) is accredited by the Accreditation Council for Continuing Medical Education (ACCME) to provide continuing medical education for physicians.

The EOCME designates this enduring material for a maximum of 15 *AMA PRA Category 1 Credit*(s)™. Physicians should claim only the credit commensurate with the extent of their participation in the activity.

All other health care professionals requesting continuing education credit for this enduring material will be issued a certificate of participation.

DISCLOSURE OF CONFLICTS OF INTEREST
The EOCME assesses conflict of interest with its instructors, faculty, planners, and other individuals who are in a position to control the content of CME activities. All relevant conflicts of interest that are identified are thoroughly vetted by EOCME for fair balance, scientific objectivity, and patient care recommendations. EOCME is committed to providing its learners with CME activities that promote improvements or quality in healthcare and not a specific proprietary business or a commercial interest.

The planning committee, staff, authors and editors listed below have identified no financial relationships or relationships to products or devices they or their spouse/life partner have with commercial interest related to the content of this CME activity:
Philippe F. Backeljauw, MD; Andrew J. Bauer, MD; Monika Chaudhari, MD; Diva D. De León, MD, MSCE; Siri Atma W. Greeley, MD, PhD; Kerry Holland; Lucky Jain, MD, MBA; Heidi E. Karpen, MD; Michelle Blanco Lemelman, MD; Lisa Letourneau, MPH, RD, LDN; Leah Logan, MBA; Katherine Lord, MD; Andrew B. Muir, MD; Sisi M. Namoc, MD; John S. Parks, MD, PhD; Jacob M. Redel, MD; Susan R. Rose, MD, MEd; Stephanie L. Samuels, MD; Susan M. Scott, MD, JD; Jonathan L. Slaughter, MD, MPH; Constantine A. Stratakis, MD, D(Med)Sc; Christina Tatsi, MD, PhD; Subhalakshmi Vaidyanathan; Ari J. Wassner, MD.

UNAPPROVED/OFF-LABEL USE DISCLOSURE
The EOCME requires CME faculty to disclose to the participants:
1. When products or procedures being discussed are off-label, unlabelled, experimental, and/or investigational (not US Food and Drug Administration [FDA] approved); and
2. Any limitations on the information presented, such as data that are preliminary or that represent ongoing research, interim analyses, and/or unsupported opinions. Faculty may discuss information about pharmaceutical agents that is outside of FDA-approved labelling. This information is intended solely for CME and is not intended to promote off-label use of these medications. If you have any questions, contact the medical affairs department of the manufacturer for the most recent prescribing information.

TO ENROLL
To enroll in the *Clinics in Perinatology* Continuing Medical Education program, call customer service at 1-800-654-2452 or sign up online at http://www.theclinics.com/home/cme. The CME program is available to subscribers for an additional annual fee of $244 USD.

METHOD OF PARTICIPATION
In order to claim credit, participants must complete the following:
1. Complete enrolment as indicated above.
2. Read the activity.

3. Complete the CME Test and Evaluation. Participants must achieve a score of 70% on the test. All CME Tests and Evaluations must be completed online.

CME INQUIRIES/SPECIAL NEEDS

For all CME inquiries or special needs, please contact elsevierCME@elsevier.com.

Endocrinology

CLINICS IN PERINATOLOGY

Foreword

Hormonal Regulation of Human Development

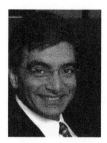

Lucky Jain, MD, MBA
Consulting Editor

The fact that hormones play a crucial and multidimensional role in physiologic processes has been evident to clinicians for a long time. The specific role hormones play in early organ development and maturation is of particular importance to neonatologists and perinatologists. While we have come a long way in eliminating preventable causes of disability of endocrine origin such as cretinism, ill effects of milder forms of altered hormonal milieu are less well understood. Indeed, when normal fetal development is interrupted by premature birth or other maternal-fetal conditions, we have learned to manage these issues largely by deduction from postnatal data.

The impact of maternal hormonal conditions, and medications used to treat them, on fetal health and well-being cannot be overstated. Yet, there is paucity of studies designed to fine-tune dosage and duration of therapy specifically from a fetal perspective. For example, let's take the landmark study by Liggins and colleagues in 1972.[1] More than 40 years after a chance application of two potent steroidal compounds to enhance fetal lung maturation was used in a randomized controlled trial, we still use the same combination of drugs and dosage employed in the original study regardless of the scaled risk of preterm birth, gestational age at treatment, and/or fetal condition. We do know that multiple courses of this potent steroid treatment can have devastating effects on the developing central nervous system.[2] Can we use a lower dose of betamethasone in certain situations? Will a single dose suffice in late-preterm gestations? Such considerations are particularly important since the indications for steroid use have expanded considerably over the years. Similarly, the incidence of congenital hypothyroidism has more than doubled in recent years due to factors that are not completely understood (**Fig. 1**).[3] The identification of IGSF1 as a cause of central congenital hypothyroidism sheds new light on regulatory pathways in multiple hormonal systems and the possibility that interplay within multiple genes may be responsible for the observed phenotype (**Fig. 2**).[4] In the absence of reliable norms for physiologic

Clin Perinatol 45 (2018) xiii–xv
https://doi.org/10.1016/j.clp.2017.12.001
0095-5108/18/© 2017 Published by Elsevier Inc.

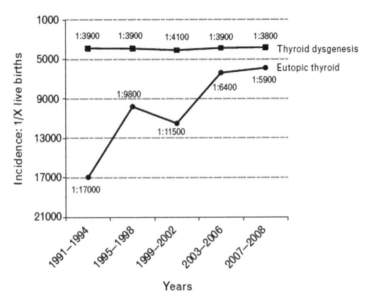

Fig. 1. The rising incidence of congenital hypothyroidism. (*From* Wassner AJ, Brown RS. Congenital hypothyroidism: recent advances. Curr Opin Endocrinol Diabetes Obes 2015;22:408; with permission.)

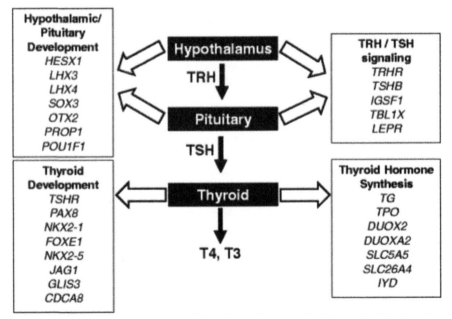

Fig. 2. Genes associated with congenital hypothyroidism. T3, triiodothyronine; T4, thyroxine; TRH, thyrotropin-releasing hormone; TSH, thyroid-stimulating hormone. (*From* Cherella CE, Wassner AJ. Congenital hypothyroidism: insights into pathogenesis and treatment. Int J Pediatr Endocrinol 2017;2017:2; with permission.)

levels and therapeutic targets, it is important to note that excess hormone treatment may be as, or even more, harmful than the underlying condition itself.

These and many other important endocrine issues have been addressed in this issue of *Clinics in Perinatology*. Drs Muir and Rose are to be congratulated for bringing to us this very timely collection of articles on a topic that is not always at the top of our priority list. As always, I am thankful to the team at Elsevier led by Kerry Holland and Casey Potter for their support, and to you, our readers, for the opportunity to represent you on the editorial team for *Clinics in Perinatology*.

Lucky Jain, MD, MBA
Department of Pediatrics
Emory University School of Medicine and
Children's Healthcare of Atlanta
2015 Uppergate Drive
Atlanta, GA 30322, USA

E-mail address:
ljain@emory.edu

REFERENCES

1. Liggins GC, Howie RN. A controlled trial of antepartum glucocorticoid treatment for prevention of the respiratory distress syndrome in premature infants. Pediatrics 1972;50(4):515–25.
2. Walfisch A, Hallak M, Mazor M. Multiple courses of antenatal steroids: risks and benefits. Obstet Gynecol 2001;98:491–7.
3. Wassner AJ, Brown RS. Congenital hypothyroidism: recent advances. Curr Opin Endocrinol Diabetes Obes 2015;22:407–12.
4. Cherella CE, Wassner AJ. Congenital hypothyroidism: insights into pathogenesis and treatment. Int J Pediatr Endocrinol 2017;2017:11.

Preface

Perinatal Endocrine Challenges

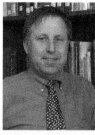 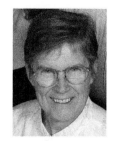

Andrew B. Muir, MD   Susan R. Rose, MD, MEd
Editors

The maturing endocrine system in preterm and full-term neonates presents diagnostic and therapeutic challenges for perinatologists and pediatricians. This issue of *Clinics in Perinatology* therefore presents reviews that outline physiologically based approaches to managing disorders of endocrinology which occur in the prenatal and early life period. With nothing less than the long-term health and development of their patients at stake, clinicians are called on to distinguish among normal immature and transitional endocrine function, fetal and neonatal reactions to maternally-derived transplacental stimuli, hormonal responses to systemic illness, medication-induced dysfunction, and true endocrine pathology. The simultaneous occurrence of many of these conditions complicates the challenge.

Frequently, disagreement over the definition of "normal" further confounds decision making in perinatal endocrine care. What is a normal blood glucose concentration during and after the birth transition? What is a normal serum cortisol concentration in response to stress?

The physiologic stresses surrounding the transition from prenatal to postnatal environment are many and can have long-term influence on health. In addition, altered fetal/ prenatal environment and nutrition leading to small-for-gestational-age or large-for-gestational-age birth weight have consequences for later life-long disease, specifically, obesity, hypertension, metabolic syndrome, and risk for type 2 diabetes and heart disease.[1–4] Even maternal nutrition prior to and during pregnancy affects the life-long health of the offspring.[5]

Today most of the difficult decisions relating to endocrine care are made after the child has arrived in the nursery. Dilemmas reviewed in this issue of *Clinics in Perinatology* include diagnosis and management of the following: congenital hypothyroidism, thyroid function in the neonatal intensive care unit (NICU), neonatal thyrotoxicosis, neonatal diabetes, hypoglycemia in association with hyperinsulinism, congenital hypopituitarism, adrenal insufficiency and glucocorticoid use in the NICU, neonatal Cushing

Clin Perinatol 45 (2018) xvii–xviii
https://doi.org/10.1016/j.clp.2017.11.004
0095-5108/18/© 2017 Published by Elsevier Inc.

disease, early identification of Turner syndrome, and bone mineral/calcium disorders in the newborn.

Discussions of the fetal diagnosis and treatment of congenital thyroid disease, congenital adrenal hyperplasia, and other issues reviewed in this issue may presage an era in which the most reliable diagnostics and safest treatments are addressed in prenatal life (Appendices A–C).

We appreciate that Dr Paul Hofman was willing to share slides from his talk at the 2017 International Pediatric Endocrine Meeting in Washington, DC.

Andrew B. Muir, MD
Pediatric Endocrinology
Emory University
Atlanta, GA 30322, USA

Susan R. Rose, MD, MEd
Pediatrics and Pediatric Endocrinology
Cincinnati Children's Hospital Medical Center
University of Cincinnati College of Medicine
MLC 7012, 3333 Burnet Avenue
Cincinnati, OH 45229, USA

E-mail addresses:
abmuir@emory.edu (A.B. Muir)
Mslrose4@gmail.com (S.R. Rose)

REFERENCES

1. Hofman PL, Cutfield WS, Robinson EM, et al. Insulin resistance in short children with intrauterine growth retardation. J Clin Endocrinol Metab 1997;82:402–6.
2. Hofman PL, Regan F, Jackson WE, et al. Premature birth and later insulin resistance. N Engl J Med 2004;8(351):2179–86.
3. Pilgaard K, Færch K, Carstensen B, et al. Low birthweight and premature birth are both associated with type 2 diabetes in a random sample of middle-aged Danes. Diabetologia 2010;53:2526–30.
4. Dabalea D, Pettitt DJ, Hanson RL, et al. Birth weight, type 2 diabetes, and insulin resistance in Pima Indian children and young adults. Diabetes Care 1999;22:944–50.
5. Whitaker RC. Predicting preschooler obesity at birth: the role of maternal obesity in early pregnancy. Pediatrics 2004;114:e29–36.

Congenital Hypothyroidism

Ari J. Wassner, MD

KEYWORDS

- Congenital hypothyroidism • Neonatal thyroid • Development • Levothyroxine
- Dysgenesis • Dyshormonogenesis

KEY POINTS

- Thyroid hormone is critical for neurodevelopment, and congenital hypothyroidism can lead to severe neurocognitive impairment.
- Most congenital hypothyroidism is caused by thyroid dysgenesis, of which the underlying causes are poorly understood; a minority of patients have a normally placed thyroid gland, while rare patients have central congenital hypothyroidism.
- Universal newborn screening is a valuable but imperfect tool for diagnosis of congenital hypothyroidism; clinical judgment and repeat screening are important in high-risk infants.
- Careful evaluation usually reveals the etiology of congenital hypothyroidism, which may inform treatment and prognosis.
- Prompt diagnosis and treatment with adequate doses of levothyroxine lead to excellent neurodevelopmental outcomes in most patients with congenital hypothyroidism.

INTRODUCTION

Thyroid hormone has important effects on almost every organ system and plays a crucial role in normal growth and neurologic development. Congenital hypothyroidism affects nearly 1 in 2000 newborns and can have devastating effects on neurocognitive development if not detected and treated early and effectively. Although the introduction of universal newborn screening has nearly eliminated congenital hypothyroidism as a cause of severe neurologic impairment in the developed world, it remains a leading cause of preventable intellectual disability in areas of the world where access to prompt diagnosis or treatment is not available. An understanding of the pathophysiology of congenital hypothyroidism and of the principles and pitfalls of newborn screening are required to appropriately identify, evaluate, and treat this condition in the newborn period. Optimal diagnosis and therapy of congenital hypothyroidism is critical to ensuring excellent outcomes, particularly in high-risk infants.

Disclosure Statement: The author has no conflicts of interest.
Thyroid Program, Division of Endocrinology, Boston Children's Hospital, Harvard Medical School, 300 Longwood Avenue, Boston, MA 02115, USA
E-mail address: ari.wassner@childrens.harvard.edu

Clin Perinatol 45 (2018) 1–18
https://doi.org/10.1016/j.clp.2017.10.004   **perinatology.theclinics.com**

THYROID PHYSIOLOGY
Function and Regulation of the Thyroid

The primary function of the thyroid gland is to produce and secrete thyroid hormones, which exert important physiologic effects throughout the body. Thyroxine (T4), the predominant hormone produced by the thyroid, is a prohormone that is converted in peripheral tissues to the biologically active hormone triiodothyronine (T3), which has a 15-fold greater affinity for the thyroid hormone receptor than T4. Most circulating T3 (80%) is derived from peripheral conversion of T4, and the remaining 20% is secreted directly from the thyroid. In the serum, both T4 and T3 are bound tightly to serum proteins including T4-binding globulin (TBG), albumin, and prealbumin, and only the tiny fraction of T4 (0.02%) and T3 (0.3%) that exists in the unbound or "free" state is able to enter cells and exert its biological actions.

The function of the thyroid gland is regulated by thyroid-stimulating hormone (TSH), which is secreted by thyrotrope cells in the anterior pituitary. Binding of TSH to its receptor on the thyroid follicular cell stimulates the synthesis and secretion of thyroid hormone, as well as growth of the thyroid gland. The production of TSH by pituitary thyrotropes is stimulated, in turn, by thyrotropin-releasing hormone (TRH), which is produced by specific neurons in the hypothalamus. Circulating thyroid hormones inhibit the secretion of both TRH and TSH, completing a negative feedback loop that maintains normal thyroid homeostasis.

Congenital hypothyroidism is an inborn condition in which the thyroid gland does not produce sufficient thyroid hormone to meet the body's needs. The causes of congenital hypothyroidism can be divided into those that directly impair thyroidal synthesis of thyroid hormone (primary hypothyroidism) and those that disrupt hypothalamic or pituitary control of the thyroid gland by decreasing the secretion and/or bioactivity of TSH (central hypothyroidism). Primary hypothyroidism is far more common than central hypothyroidism.

In primary hypothyroidism, the hypothalamus and pituitary respond appropriately to decreased thyroidal production of thyroid hormones by increasing the serum concentration of TSH. Because TSH increases significantly in responses to small changes in serum free T4 (FT4) levels, TSH is the most sensitive test for primary hypothyroidism, and in mild cases the serum TSH becomes elevated before FT4 concentrations fall below normal. In central hypothyroidism, serum concentrations of thyroid hormones are low, but owing to the hypothalamic or pituitary defect, serum levels of TSH do not increase appropriately, but instead remain normal or low.

Fetal Thyroid Development and Physiology

The fetal thyroid gland begins to form about 3 weeks after conception as a thickening of cells (thyroid anlage) in the floor of the primitive pharynx, at what will become the base of the tongue (foramen cecum). The anlage forms a thyroid bud that descends caudally over the next few weeks to its final position in the anterior neck. During this descent, the connection to the pharynx (thyroglossal duct) is normally obliterated, although remnants can persist and cause thyroglossal duct cysts. By week 10 of gestation, the fetal thyroid is able to trap iodide and synthesize thyroid hormones; however, hypothalamic and pituitary control is not established until the second trimester, and the axis continues to mature throughout the third trimester.

Thyroid hormone plays a critical role in brain development beginning in the first trimester and through the first few years of life. Hypothyroidism during this period can have devastating neurodevelopmental consequences.[1,2] During the first trimester, before the onset of fetal thyroid hormone synthesis, the embryo is completely dependent for normal development on maternal T4, which passes in limited amounts across the placenta.[3] Transplacental passage of maternal T4 continues through the third trimester and accounts for a significant proportion of fetal T4 until birth. This transfer, along with changes in thyroid hormone metabolism, serves to protect the developing brain from thyroid hormone deficiency, even in fetuses with severe congenital hypothyroidism. For this reason, problems causing concurrent maternal and fetal hypothyroidism (such as iodine deficiency or TSH receptor blocking anti-bodies) may have more profound detrimental effects on fetal neurodevelopment than does isolated fetal hypothyroidism.[4]

EPIDEMIOLOGY

When newborn screening for congenital hypothyroidism was introduced in the 1970s, the incidence of this condition was about 1 in 4000 infants.[5] Over the past several de-cades, however, the apparent incidence of congenital hypothyroidism has nearly doubled, with studies from multiple countries—including Greece, the United States, Canada, New Zealand, Argentina, and Italy—reporting incidence rates between 1 in 1400 and 1 in 2800.[6–11] Several factors likely account for this change. The most impor-tant factor is the lowering of TSH screening cutoffs that has occurred in many newborn screening programs, which has led to increased detection of milder cases of congen-ital hypothyroidism. In contrast, the incidence of severe congenital hypothyroidism has remained unchanged over this period.[7,8,11] Changing demographics may also in-fluence the apparent incidence of this disorder. For example, 1 study demonstrated that the increase in incidence from 1 in 3846 to 1 in 2778 observed in New Zealand over 17 years was attributable to an increase in birth rates among Asians and Pacific Islanders, ethnic groups that are at increased risk of congenital hypothyroidism.[9] A similar phenomenon has been observed in the United States with the increase in the Hispanic population, another group at increased risk.[12] A final possible factor is the increasing number and survival of preterm and low birth weight (LBW) infants due to improvements in neonatal intensive care. Although LBW infants are at higher risk of congenital hypothyroidism, studies from Quebec and Massachusetts indicate that they likely account for no more than a small fraction of its increasing incidence.[7,8]

CAUSES OF CONGENITAL HYPOTHYROIDISM
Primary Congenital Hypothyroidism

Primary defects of the thyroid gland can be caused by failure of normal thyroid devel-opment (thyroid dysgenesis) or by failure of an anatomically normal (eutopic) thyroid gland to produce sufficient thyroid hormone (dyshormonogenesis). The majority of congenital hypothyroidism is caused by thyroid dysgenesis. Dysgenesis encom-passes a spectrum of phenotypes, including complete thyroid agenesis, aberrant migration resulting in a (dysfunctional) ectopic gland, and a normally placed but hypo-plastic thyroid. Thyroid dysgenesis is usually sporadic, and the underlying cause of most cases remains unknown. In a minority of cases (2–5%), a mutation may be pre-sent in one of several genes involved in thyroid gland formation, including the TSH re-ceptor (*TSHR*) or the transcription factors *PAX8*, *NKX2-1*, or *FOXE1*.[13] More recently, several additional genes have been associated with thyroid dysgenesis, including *NKX2-5*,[14,15] *JAG1*,[16] and *GLIS3*,[17] although each likely contributes to only a small fraction of cases. Each of these transcription factors has developmental roles in other organ systems, and mutations are generally associated with additional congenital de-fects (**Table 1**). Although the number of genes associated with thyroid dysgenesis continues to increase, it is not clear that a significant proportion of cases will be

Table 1
Clinical features of genetic syndromes associated with thyroid dysgenesis

Gene	Associated Abnormalities
PAX8	Urogenital abnormalities
NKX2-1	Interstitial lung disease, chorea
FOXE1	Cleft palate, bifid epiglottis, choanal atresia, spiky hair (Bamforth-Lazarus syndrome)
NKX2-5	Congenital heart disease
JAG1	Alagille syndrome (variable liver, heart, eye, skeletal, facial defects), congenital heart disease
GLIS3	Neonatal diabetes mellitus, developmental delay, congenital glaucoma, hepatic fibrosis, polycystic kidneys

explained by germline genetic mutations, given the fact that monozygotic twins—who share an identical germline genetic complement—are frequently discordant for thyroid dysgenesis.[18]

Although thyroid dysgenesis is the most common cause of primary congenital hypothyroidism, its incidence (about 1 in 4000) has remained steady over the last 25 years, whereas the incidence of dyshormonogenesis has increased sharply.[19] As a result, patients with a eutopic thyroid now account for 30% to 40% of congenital hypothyroidism, compared with only around 15% in the early days of newborn screening.[8,11] Dyshormonogenesis is often caused by mutations in genes that encode the cellular machinery of thyroid hormone synthesis, including the sodium-iodide symporter (NIS; SLC5A5), the apical iodide transporter pendrin (PDS; SLC26A4), thyroperoxidase (TPO), thyroglobulin (TG), dual oxidase 2 (DUOX2) and its accessory protein (DUOXA2), and iodotyrosine deiodinase (IYD; **Fig. 1**).[20] Recent studies suggest that 50% or more of patient with a eutopic thyroid may carry variants in at least 1, and frequently 2 or more, of these genes.[21–23]

Neonatal hypothyroidism with a eutopic thyroid gland can also be caused by a number of factors extrinsic to the thyroid gland. Antithyroid drugs (methimazole or propylthiouracil) given during pregnancy to treat maternal hyperthyroidism are transported across the placenta and can cause transient congenital hypothyroidism until the drug is clear from the infant's circulation (about 7–10 days). In infants of mothers with autoimmune thyroid disease (including Graves' disease), immunoglobulin G antibodies that block activation of the TSH receptor can cross the placenta and cause similar transient hypothyroidism that may require 3 to 6 months to resolve.

Because iodine is an essential constituent of thyroid hormone, iodine deficiency is an important cause of congenital hypothyroidism worldwide, particularly in iodine-deficient areas where salt iodization programs have not been implemented. Preterm infants are at increased risk of iodine deficiency, in part because parenteral nutrition and preterm infant formulas commonly used in intensive care settings may provide inadequate iodine.[24] Excess iodine intake normally causes a physiologic decrease in thyroid hormone synthesis (the Wolff-Chaikoff effect) that is usually transient.[25] However, because the thyroid's ability to recover (or "escape") from this effect does not mature until 36 to 40 weeks of gestation, preterm infants are at risk of prolonged hypothyroidism from exposure to excess iodine. Excess iodine may derive from iodine-containing antiseptics,[26,27] radiographic contrast agents,[28] or copious maternal intake of iodine (from diet or supplements) that is transmitted to the infant in breastmilk.[29,30]

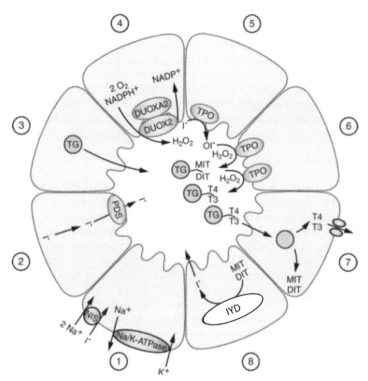

Fig. 1. Thyroid hormone synthesis. (1) Iodide is transported into the cell by the sodium–iodide symporter (NIS; *SLC5A5*). This step depends on the generation of an electrochemical gradient generated by the Na^+/K^+-ATPase. (2) Iodide is transported into the follicular lumen, at least in part by pendrin (PDS; *SLC26A4*). (3) Thyroglobulin (TG) is secreted into the follicular lumen, where it serves as the matrix for the synthesis of thyroxine (T4) and triiodothyronine (T3). (4) The oxidation of iodide requires hydrogen peroxide (H_2O_2) generated by the dual oxidase DUOX2, an enzyme that requires the maturation factor DUOXA2 for normal function. (5) Iodide is oxidized by the enzyme thyroperoxidase (TPO). (6) TPO iodinates selected tyrosine residues on TG to form monoiodotyrosines (MIT) and diiodotyrosines (DIT). The iodotyrosines are then coupled by TPO to form T4 or T3. (7) Iodinated TG is internalized by endocytosis and digested in lysosomes, and T4 and T3 are secreted into the circulation. (8) Residual MIT and DIT are deiodinated in the cytosol by iodotyrosine deiodinase (IYD), and the released iodide is recycled for thyroid hormone synthesis. (*Adapted from* Kopp P, Solis JC. Thyroid hormone synthesis. In: Wondisford FE, Radovick S, editors. Clinical management of thyroid disease. Philadelphia: Saunders; 2009. p. 20; with permission.)

Central Congenital Hypothyroidism

Central congenital hypothyroidism is rare, and early studies estimated its incidence between 1 in 29,000 and 1 in 110,000 newborns.[5,31] However, more recent data from the Netherlands using a rigorous newborn screening strategy indicate that the incidence of central congenital hypothyroidism may be as high as 1 in 16,000.[32,33] Inborn central defects of the thyroid axis are usually due to structural or developmental abnormalities of the hypothalamus or pituitary. Such defects tend to affect additional pituitary hormone axes (growth hormone, prolactin, adrenocorticotropin, gonadotropins), and deficiencies of multiple pituitary hormones are present in about 75% of newborns with central hypothyroidism.[33] Some of these cases are due to genetic mutations in transcription factors involved in hypothalamic or pituitary development such as *HESX1*, *LHX3*, *LHX4*, *OTX2*, *SOX3*, *PROP1*, and *POU1F1*.[34] Rarely, central congenital hypothyroidism may be caused by specific genetic defects in TRH or TSH signaling. The most common of these is an inactivating mutation in the recently described X-linked gene *IGSF1*,[35] which encodes a cell surface glycoprotein that seems to promote normal expression of the TRH receptor in pituitary thyrotropes.[36,37] Other very rare genetic causes include mutations in the TRH receptor itself (*TRHR*),[38] the β-subunit of TSH (*TSHB*),[39] and another X-linked gene, *TBL1X*.[40] Central hypothyroidism can also occur (usually transiently) in infants exposed to maternal hyperthyroidism during pregnancy.

CLINICAL MANIFESTATIONS

Aside from its crucial role in neurodevelopment and growth, thyroid hormone has important effects on many other organ systems. In the cardiovascular system, thyroid hormone decreases systemic vascular resistance and increases cardiac rate, contractility, and output. It also promotes renal excretion of salt and water, stimulates gastrointestinal motility, and increases the basal metabolic rate and body temperature. Symptoms and signs of congenital hypothyroidism, shown in **Box 1**, reflect the absence of these normal thyroid hormone effects. However, it is important to recognize that these symptoms and signs are nonspecific and can be observed in many other neonatal illnesses. Furthermore, obvious clinical manifestations of hypothyroidism are usually absent in newborns—even those with severe hypothyroidism—which reinforces the central role of universal newborn screening in facilitating prompt diagnosis and treatment. In contrast, like all tests, newborn screening is subject to errors and false-negative results, so practitioners must have a low threshold to evaluate for hypothyroidism in any infant with suggestive findings regardless of prior newborn screening results. In particular, the presence of goiter, poor linear growth, prolonged indirect hyperbilirubinemia, or a widened posterior fontanelle (>0.5 cm) should raise suspicion for possible congenital hypothyroidism.

About 10% of infants with congenital hypothyroidism have other congenital abnormalities, the most common of which are cardiac defects. Thyroid hormone plays an important role in cochlear development, and hearing loss of varying severity also

| Box 1 |
Symptoms and signs of congenital hypothyroidism in infants
Goiter
Poor feeding
Constipation
Hypothermia
Bradycardia
Edema
Large fontanelles
Macroglossia
Prolonged jaundice
Umbilical hernia
Poor growth
Developmental delay

occurs in up to 10% of patients with congenital hypothyroidism by early adulthood.[41] Finally, genetic causes of congenital hypothyroidism are associated with specific syndromic features, which include urogenital anomalies, such as unilateral renal agenesis and horseshoe kidney (PAX8); interstitial lung disease and chorea (NKX2-1); cleft palate, bifid epiglottis, and spiky hair (FOXE1); Alagille syndrome (JAG1); and neonatal diabetes, congenital glaucoma, and liver and kidney abnormalities (GLIS3; see **Table 1**).[42]

DIAGNOSIS

Universal newborn screening is the most important tool for diagnosing congenital hypothyroidism and is practiced routinely in most of the developed world. Specific screening practices vary by region, but in general begin in the first few days of life with collection of a heel-prick blood sample on a filter paper card that is sent to a central laboratory for analysis. Most screening programs around the world measure the blood concentration of TSH; in some programs, T4 is also measured routinely, or by reflex if the TSH is elevated.[43] This TSH-based strategy is sensitive for detecting primary hypothyroidism, including mild cases in which TSH is elevated but T4 levels remain normal. However, this strategy will not detect patients with central hypothyroidism, in whom the TSH is (by definition) not increased despite low T4 levels.

Some newborn screening programs begin by measuring T4, with reflex measurement of TSH in patients with low T4 levels. This strategy has the advantage that it may detect central hypothyroidism, although its sensitivity for this condition is variable depending on the precise strategy used. For example, the Netherlands has a robust T4-based strategy that reliably detects central hypothyroidism by collecting samples at 4 to 7 days of age, measuring TSH in infants whose TSH is in the lowest 20%, and measuring TBG in infants whose T4 is in the lowest 5%.[32,33] In contrast, a study from Indiana found that only 19% of infants with confirmed central hypothyroidism were detected base on low T4 levels (<5 mcg/dL) on newborn screening.[44] T4-based screening strategies also detect patients with X-linked congenital deficiency of TBG, a benign variant that results in low levels of total T4 but normal FT4 and TSH. Affected male patients are euthyroid and should not be treated, so they must be distinguished from patients with true central hypothyroidism who do require treatment.

The optimal time to collect a screening blood sample is between 48 and 72 hours of life, but many screening programs extend this window to 24 hours of life to capture the large number of healthy term infants discharged early from the hospital.[45] The rationale for delaying sampling beyond 48 hours of life is the physiologic surge of TSH secretion that occurs in the first hours after birth to a mean peak serum level of 80 mIU/L, which slowly decreases over the next several days.[46] Therefore, blood samples obtained too early (particularly in the first 24 hours of life) may yield false positives in TSH-based screens. Nevertheless, in certain situations (such as in infants who require blood transfusion or transfer to another unit or facility), it is preferable to obtain a screening sample early rather than to forgo the opportunity to screen entirely.

Despite its high sensitivity, newborn screening in the first days of life is not perfect and may have up to a 10% false-negative rate.[47] There are several important causes of false-negative screening results. First, in some patients with primary congenital hypothyroidism, the increase in serum TSH is delayed and may not occur for several weeks. This pattern is particularly common in preterm or very LBW infants (<1500 g). Although these infants have a 14-fold greater risk of congenital hypothyroidism than normal weight infants, around two-thirds of cases may manifest a delayed TSH increase, which may occur in as many as 1 in 85 very LBW infants.[7,48,49] A similar effect may be seen in infants admitted to neonatal intensive care units owing to illness and/or drugs used to treat them (eg, dopamine, glucocorticoids). Monozygotic twins are another group at risk of false-negative screening. Although they are frequently discordant for congenital hypothyroidism,[18] if twins share a placental circulation, the normal twin's thyroid may compensate in utero for the hypothyroid twin. Because T4 has a relatively long half-life (3–4 days in the neonate),[3] the hypothyroid twin may not be detected on initial newborn screening and may present later with untreated hypothyroidism. Finally, technical or human errors in screening can result in some infants with congenital hypothyroidism going undetected. False-positive results are also more common in preterm and LBW infants.[50]

To address some of these potential issues, repeat newborn screening at 2 to 4 weeks of age should be considered in patients at risk of false-negative screening, including preterm and LBW infants, critically ill infants, same-sex twins, and infants whose initial screen was performed in the first 24 hours of life.[45] Repeat screening should also be considered for other infants at increased risk of hypothyroidism, including those with trisomy 21 and those at risk of iodine excess or iodine deficiency. Some newborn screening programs require such repeat screening for some or all of these categories of infants, and a few programs routinely perform second screens on all newborns.[51]

MANAGEMENT AND PROGNOSIS
Management of Abnormal Newborn Screening Results

Any abnormal result on newborn screening should prompt immediate confirmation (ideally within 24 hours) by measuring serum concentrations of TSH and FT4. It is important to be aware that some laboratories may report TSH and FT4 reference ranges that are not applicable to infants, so all results should be interpreted based on gestational age- and postnatal age-specific reference ranges.[52] It is also important to account for the administration of medications that can affect thyroid hormone assays, such as heparin, furosemide, fatty acids, or biotin. In general, a pediatric endocrinologist should be enlisted as soon as possible to assist with the evaluation and possible treatment of any patient with suspected congenital hypothyroidism.

Infants in whom the TSH is elevated on newborn screening have primary hypothyroidism, and the severity of the hypothyroidism determines the urgency of treatment. If the newborn screening TSH is greater than 40 mIU/L, severe hypothyroidism should be presumed and treatment should be initiated as soon as confirmatory serum laboratory tests are drawn, without waiting for the results. Once confirmatory measurements are available, treatment should be initiated in any patient with a serum TSH of greater than 20 mIU/L, or with a low FT4 concentration regardless of TSH concentration.[45]

Infants with a slight elevation of TSH and normal FT4 levels have mild hypothyroidism, and current data are indeterminate as to the neurodevelopmental risks posed by this degree of hypothyroidism and whether treatment is of benefit. A series of recent studies of Belgian children showed no association between mild TSH elevation on newborn screening and cognitive or psychomotor development at preschool age.[53,54] In contrast, a population-based study of more than 500,000 Australian children demonstrated a positive association between increasing newborn screening TSH concentrations of up to 12 to 14 mIU/L, and an increased risk of adverse developmental or educational outcomes.[55] Both studies have limitations, however, and the true risk posed by mild congenital hypothyroidism remains unclear. For patients with confirmatory serum TSH levels of 6 to 20 mIU/L and normal FT4 levels, it is reasonable to follow serum thyroid function tests closely (every 1–2 weeks) and to initiate treatment if TSH is increasing or if FT4 decreases to below normal. When such mild hypothyroidism persists for more than 3 to 4 weeks, consensus recommendations indicate that further observation may be considered, but also acknowledge the inclination of many clinicians to initiate treatment in an effort to avoid potential (but unproven) neurodevelopmental risks.[45]

In infants with primary hypothyroidism, additional evaluation may help to establish the cause and potentially inform treatment and/or prognosis. Thyroid imaging (either by ultrasound or scintigraphy) may establish a diagnosis of thyroid dysgenesis, which is likely to be permanent and therefore requires treatment even if mild. In contrast, the presence of a eutopic thyroid gland suggests the possibility of transient hypothyroidism. In several studies that collectively evaluated 159 patients with a eutopic thyroid gland around 3 years of age, 35% were found to have transient congenital hypothyroidism that had resolved.[19,56–58] Interestingly, the likelihood of transient hypothyroidism was not related to the initial severity of TSH elevation,[56] which highlights the importance of offering a trial off therapy at 3 years of age for these patients. Importantly, however, if treatment is indicated, it should never be delayed by plans for imaging.

In addition to radiographic studies, measurement of serum thyroglobulin levels can provide useful information about the etiology of congenital hypothyroidism. Thyroglobulin is synthesized by thyroid follicular cells and its production is stimulated by activation of the TSH receptor, so the serum concentration of thyroglobulin reflects the body's functional thyroid mass. When measured at a time of elevated TSH concentrations, a low level of thyroglobulin indicates reduced thyroid mass (ie, dysgenesis), a rare mutation of the thyroglobulin gene, or impaired function of the TSH receptor itself, which may be caused by genetic defects in TSH receptor signaling or by maternal TSH receptor-blocking antibodies. The latter is important to diagnose because it portends a transient course of hypothyroidism that will resolve within a few months. Therefore, the presence of a normal thyroid gland on anatomic imaging (ultrasound) combined with a low serum thyroglobulin concentration should prompt testing for TSH receptor antibodies. The presence of such antibodies should also be considered in any infant with congenital hypothyroidism and a maternal history of autoimmune thyroid disease, although absence of such a maternal history is not sufficient to exclude this possibility.[4]

Infants with low T4 and normal TSH on newborn screening present a differential diagnosis distinct from those with primary hypothyroidism. If the patient is male and confirmatory testing shows normal FT4 levels, TBG deficiency may be present and can be confirmed by measuring the serum concentration of TBG. If serum FT4 is low on confirmatory testing, the possibility of central hypothyroidism must be considered. Other signs of hypopituitarism should be sought, including midline defects, hypoglycemia, direct hyperbilirubinemia, diabetes insipidus, or microphallus or undescended testes in a male infant. Further evaluation may include MRI of the pituitary and hypothalamus and laboratory assessment of pituitary hormone function. Formal examination of the optic discs may reveal evidence of septooptic dysplasia. Proper diagnosis of central hypothyroidism is essential because associated untreated adrenal insufficiency or growth hormone deficiency can be life threatening.

The evaluation of infants with low FT4 and normal TSH should also take account of gestational age and birth weight. This pattern of thyroid function may be present in up to 50% of preterm and LBW infants and has been termed hypothyroxinemia of prematurity.[59] The pathogenesis of this condition is multifactorial and includes premature withdrawal of maternal thyroid hormone, immaturity of the hypothalamic–pituitary–thyroid axis, changes in thyroid hormone metabolism, the often serious illnesses frequently present in these infants and some of the medications used to treat them. The clinical significance and appropriate management of hypothyroxinemia of prematurity remain uncertain and are discussed in greater detail in the Monika Chaudhari and Jonathan L. Slaughter's article, "Thyroid Function in the Neonatal Intensive Care Unit," in this issue.

Levothyroxine Treatment and Monitoring

Levothyroxine (LT4) is the treatment for congenital hypothyroidism. Alternative thyroid medications, including desiccated thyroid preparations and products containing T3, are not recommended.[45,60] Treatment should be started as soon as the diagnosis is confirmed, ideally within the first 2 weeks of life. The recommended starting dose is 10 to 15 mg/kg, and within this range the dose may be individualized based on the severity of hypothyroidism. Late initiation of treatment and lower initial doses of LT4 are associated with poorer neurodevelopmental outcomes.[45,60–62]

LT4 should be given in tablet form owing to the inconsistent delivery of many liquid formulations. Tablets can be crushed, mixed with a small amount (1–2 mL) of water, breast milk, or non–soy-based formula, and administered orally by syringe. LT4 should not be given with soy formula or products, which impair LT4 absorption and are a well-established cause of undertreatment of congenital hypothyroidism.[63,64] If LT4 must be given intravenously, 75% of the oral dose should be used.[65]

The goal of treatment is to achieve euthyroidism rapidly and to maintain it as consistently as possible thereafter. Normalization of serum TSH and FT4 levels within 2 weeks after starting therapy seems to improve cognitive outcomes,[62] and undertreatment in the first years of life is associated with adverse neurodevelopmental outcomes.[61,66–69] However, it is also important to avoid overtreatment with LT4, which may also be harmful.[70,71] Because the currently recommended starting dose of LT4 often leads to overtreatment,[72] careful surveillance—and often LT4 dose reduction—is necessary after initiating treatment to normalize thyroid function quickly without overtreating.

The treatment of congenital hypothyroidism is monitored by measuring serum TSH and FT4 concentrations. These should be checked 1 to 2 weeks after starting treatment and every 2 to 4 weeks thereafter, with appropriate adjustment of LT4 dose, until they have normalized. Ongoing management is focused on consistent maintenance of euthyroidism, particularly in the first 3 years of life when brain development is most dependent on thyroid hormone. Serum TSH should be maintained in the age-specific normal range, and serum FT4 should be maintained in the upper half of the age-specific normal range.[45,73–75] To achieve this goal, monitoring of serum thyroid function tests is necessary every 1 to 2 months in the first 6 months of life, every 1 to 3 months in the second 6 months, and then every 2 to 4 months through 3 years of age. TSH and FT4 should also be checked 4 weeks after any change in LT4 dose.[45]

Some patients with congenital hypothyroidism may fail to achieve normal TSH concentrations with typical (or even increased) doses of LT4. The most common reason for inadequate control is poor adherence to therapy. Therefore, adherence should be verified carefully in any patient who does not show the expected response to treatment. This verification should include reviewing the method of LT4 administration and evaluating for possible impaired absorption of LT4 owing to gastrointestinal conditions (eg, celiac disease) or co-administration of substances that may impair LT4 absorption (eg, soy formula, calcium, or iron supplements). It is also critical to ensure that the family understands the importance of adequate treatment to optimize outcomes. When TSH concentrations are increased in the setting of high-normal or elevated serum FT4, possible explanations include measurement within 4 hours of an LT4 dose (when FT4 concentrations are increased) or chronic poor adherence to therapy followed by "making up" multiple doses shortly before thyroid function is checked. However, even with optimal adherence and thyroid function assessment, some children with congenital hypothyroidism require unusually high LT4 doses and serum FT4 concentrations to normalize their TSH. This phenomenon reflects a degree of resistance to T4 action at the hypothalamic or pituitary level that may occur in up to 40% of infants with congenital hypothyroidism, and usually improves over time.[76] The mechanism underlying this resistance is unknown, but may relate to effects of mild fetal hypothyroidism on the development of the hypothalamic–pituitary–thyroid axis. In such patients, T4 resistance may make it difficult or impossible to achieve TSH and FT4 simultaneously within the reference range, as recommended in current consensus guidelines. No outcome-based evidence exists to guide optimal management of such patients, but it seems reasonable to attempt to achieve a combination of TSH and FT4 levels each as close to the reference range as possible while avoiding marked elevations of either.

Prognosis

The primary concern for families of infants diagnosed with congenital hypothyroidism is whether their child will suffer any adverse long-term consequences from the condition. In general, developmental outcomes in congenital hypothyroidism are excellent, and early and adequate treatment with LT4 prevents severe neurocognitive deficits and results in normal global intelligence (IQ). However, mild deficits in several domains—including motor development, verbal skills, attention, and memory—may occur in some patients despite optimal postnatal treatment, particularly those born with very low serum concentrations of FT4.[1,77–79]

Another frequent concern for families is whether congenital hypothyroidism will be permanent or transient. If thyroid dysgenesis is present, lifelong treatment will be required. In contrast, a transient course can be anticipated in cases related to specific extrinsic etiologies that should resolve (eg, maternal antithyroid drugs or TSH receptor-blocking antibodies). In the remaining patients with a eutopic thyroid but no identifiable inciting cause, which patients will prove to have transient disease cannot be predicted with confidence at diagnosis. Therefore, such patients may be offered a trial off therapy after 3 years of age to determine if hypothyroidism has resolved. Patients requiring a daily LT4 dose less than 2 μg/kg at 3 years of age have a greater likelihood of successfully discontinuing treatment.[56]

SUMMARY

Congenital hypothyroidism is common and can cause severe neurodevelopmental morbidity. Prompt diagnosis and the institution of early and adequate treatment are critical to preventing these adverse effects and optimizing long-term outcomes. Universal newborn screening is an important tool for the detection of congenital hypothyroidism and has led to a dramatic reduction in severe intellectual disability owing to this condition. However, newborn screening in the first days of life has limitations. Awareness of these limitations, repeated screening in high-risk infants, and a high index of clinical suspicion are needed to ensure that all infants are appropriately diagnosed and treated. Careful evaluation, including a history, physical examination, directed laboratory investigation, and adjunctive imaging, will usually reveal the underlying cause of congenital hypothyroidism, which may inform treatment decisions and prognosis. Treatment with LT4 should be initiated as early as possible, ideally within the first 2 weeks of life, and normal thyroid function should be achieved rapidly and maintained carefully. When properly managed, patients with congenital hypothyroidism overall have an excellent prognosis, but subtle deficits may remain in patients with the most severe hypothyroidism.

Best Practices

What is the current practice?

To optimize neurodevelopmental outcomes in congenital hypothyroidism, current practices include:

- Universal newborn screening,
- Prompt evaluation of abnormal screening results and treatment with adequate doses of LT4, and
- Close monitoring of treated infants to maintain euthyroidism.

Best practices, guidelines, and care path objective(s)

- Newborn screening for congenital hypothyroidism should be performed on all infants between 24 to 72 hours of life.

- Abnormal screening results should be confirmed immediately by measuring serum TSH and FT4.

- LT4 treatment (10–15 µg/kg per day) should be given to infants with confirmatory serum TSH of 20 mIU/L or greater or low FT4. Infants with milder abnormalities may be treated or followed closely.

- Repeat screening should be performed at 2 to 4 weeks of life in infants at high risk of congenital hypothyroidism or of false-negative early screening.

What changes in current practice are likely to improve outcomes?

- Worldwide implementation of universal newborn screening, and of salt iodization programs in iodine-deficient areas.

- Avoidance, when possible, of modifiable or iatrogenic risk factors (eg, iodine excess or deficiency).

- Further research into the risks posed by mild congenital hypothyroidism and to what degree treatment is of benefit.

- Greater understanding of the effects of fetal hypothyroidism on neurodevelopment and whether prevention or treatment of fetal hypothyroidism can prevent the mild developmental abnormalities observed in some patients with congenital hypothyroidism despite optimal postnatal treatment.

Is there a clinical algorithm?

See **Fig. 2** for the current evaluation and management algorithm.

Bibliographic source(s)

- Leger J, Olivieri A, Donaldson M, et al. European Society for Paediatric Endocrinology consensus guidelines on screening, diagnosis, and management of congenital hypothyroidism. Horm Res Paediatr 2014;81(2):80–103.

- Rose SR, Brown RS, Foley T, et al. Update of newborn screening and therapy for congenital hypothyroidism. Pediatrics 2006;117(6):2290–303.

Summary statement

Congenital hypothyroidism is common and can cause severe neurodevelopmental morbidity. Prompt diagnosis and institution of early and adequate treatment are critical to preventing these adverse effects and optimizing long-term outcomes. Universal newborn screening is an important tool for the detection of congenital hypothyroidism and has led to a dramatic decrease in severe intellectual disability owing to this condition. However, newborn screening in the first days of life has limitations, and awareness of these limitations, repeated screening in high-risk infants, and a high index of clinical suspicion are needed to ensure that all infants are appropriately diagnosed and treated. Careful evaluation including the history, physical examination, directed laboratory investigation, and adjunctive imaging will usually reveal the underlying cause of congenital hypothyroidism, which may inform treatment decisions and prognosis. Treatment with LT4 should be initiated as early as possible, ideally within the first 2 weeks of life, and normal thyroid function should be achieved rapidly and maintained carefully. When managed properly, patients with congenital hypothyroidism overall have an excellent prognosis, but subtle deficits may remain in patients with the most severe hypothyroidism.

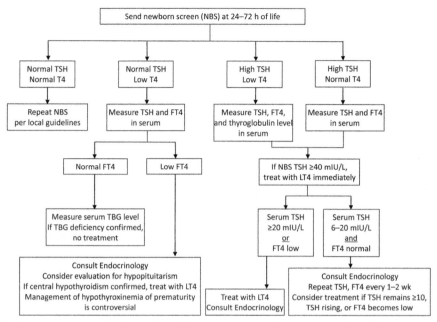

Fig. 2. Management of abnormal newborn screening results. FT4, serum free thyroxine; LT4, levothyroxine; T4, thyroxine; TBG, thyroxine-binding globulin; TSH, thyroid-stimulating hormone. (*Adapted from* Belfort MB, Brown RS. Hypothyroidism in the preterm infant. In: Brodsky D, Ouellette MA, editors. Primary care of the premature infant. Philadelphia: Saunders; 2008. p. 207–14; with permission.)

REFERENCES

1. Rovet JF. Congenital hypothyroidism: long-term outcome. Thyroid 1999;9(7): 741–8.

2. Morreale de Escobar G, Obregon MJ, Escobar del Rey F. Role of thyroid hormone during early brain development. Eur J Endocrinol 2004;151(Suppl 3): U25–37.

3. Vulsma T, Gons MH, de Vijlder JJ. Maternal-fetal transfer of thyroxine in congenital hypothyroidism due to a total organification defect or thyroid agenesis. N Engl J Med 1989;321(1):13–6.

4. Brown RS, Alter CA, Sadeghi-Nejad A. Severe unsuspected maternal hypothyroidism discovered after the diagnosis of thyrotropin receptor-blocking antibody-induced congenital hypothyroidism in the neonate: failure to recognize and implications to the fetus. Horm Res Paediatr 2015;83(2):132–5.

5. Fisher DA, Dussault JH, Foley TP Jr, et al. Screening for congenital hypothyroidism: results of screening one million North American infants. J Pediatr 1979;94(5): 700–5.

6. Mengreli C, Kanaka-Gantenbein C, Girginoudis P, et al. Screening for congenital hypothyroidism: the significance of threshold limit in false-negative results. J Clin Endocrinol Metab 2010;95(9):4283–90.

7. Mitchell ML, Hsu HW, Sahai I. The increased incidence of congenital hypothyroidism: fact or fancy? Clin Endocrinol (Oxf) 2011;75(6):806–10.

8. Deladoey J, Ruel J, Giguere Y, et al. Is the incidence of congenital hypothyroidism really increasing? A 20-year retrospective population-based study in Quebec. J Clin Endocrinol Metab 2011;96(8):2422–9.

9. Albert BB, Cutfield WS, Webster D, et al. Etiology of increasing incidence of congenital hypothyroidism in New Zealand from 1993-2010. J Clin Endocrinol Metab 2012;97(9):3155–60.

10. Chiesa A, Prieto L, Mendez V, et al. Prevalence and etiology of congenital hypothyroidism detected through an argentine neonatal screening program (1997-2010). Horm Res Paediatr 2013;80(3):185–92.

11. Olivieri A, Fazzini C, Medda E, Collaborators. Multiple factors influencing the incidence of congenital hypothyroidism detected by neonatal screening. Horm Res Paediatr 2015;83(2):86–93.

12. Hinton CF, Harris KB, Borgfeld L, et al. Trends in incidence rates of congenital hypothyroidism related to select demographic factors: data from the United States, California, Massachusetts, New York, and Texas. Pediatrics 2010;125(Suppl 2): S37–47.

13. Szinnai G. Clinical genetics of congenital hypothyroidism. Endocr Dev 2014;26: 60–78.

14. Dentice M, Cordeddu V, Rosica A, et al. Missense mutation in the transcription factor NKX2-5: a novel molecular event in the pathogenesis of thyroid dysgenesis. J Clin Endocrinol Metab 2006;91(4):1428–33.

15. Wang F, Liu C, Jia X, et al. Next-generation sequencing of NKX2.1, FOXE1, PAX8, NKX2.5, and TSHR in 100 Chinese patients with congenital hypothyroidism and athyreosis. Clin Chim Acta 2017;470:36–41.

16. de Filippis T, Marelli F, Nebbia G, et al. JAG1 loss-of-function variations as a novel predisposing event in the pathogenesis of congenital thyroid defects. J Clin Endocrinol Metab 2016;101(3):861–70.

17. Senee V, Chelala C, Duchatelet S, et al. Mutations in GLIS3 are responsible for a rare syndrome with neonatal diabetes mellitus and congenital hypothyroidism. Nat Genet 2006;38(6):682–7.

18. Perry R, Heinrichs C, Bourdoux P, et al. Discordance of monozygotic twins for thyroid dysgenesis: implications for screening and for molecular pathophysiology. J Clin Endocrinol Metab 2002;87(9):4072–7.

19. Wassner AJ, Brown RS. Congenital hypothyroidism: recent advances. Curr Opin Endocrinol Diabetes Obes 2015;22(5):407–12.

20. Grasberger H, Refetoff S. Genetic causes of congenital hypothyroidism due to dyshormonogenesis. Curr Opin Pediatr 2011;23(4):421–8.

21. Park KJ, Park HK, Kim YJ, et al. DUOX2 mutations are frequently associated with congenital hypothyroidism in the Korean population. Ann Lab Med 2016;36(2): 145–53.

22. Nicholas AK, Serra EG, Cangul H, et al. Comprehensive screening of eight known causative genes in congenital hypothyroidism with gland-in-situ. J Clin Endocrinol Metab 2016;101(12):4521–31.

23. de Filippis T, Gelmini G, Paraboschi E, et al. A frequent oligogenic involvement in congenital hypothyroidism. Hum Mol Genet 2017;26(13):2507–14.

24. Belfort MB, Pearce EN, Braverman LE, et al. Low iodine content in the diets of hospitalized preterm infants. J Clin Endocrinol Metab 2012;97(4):E632–6.

25. Wolff J, Chaikoff IL. Plasma inorganic iodide as a homeostatic regulator of thyroid function. J Biol Chem 1948;174(2):555–64.

26. Linder N, Davidovitch N, Reichman B, et al. Topical iodine-containing antiseptics and subclinical hypothyroidism in preterm infants. J Pediatr 1997;131(3):434–9.

27. Williams FL, Watson J, Day C, et al. Thyroid dysfunction in preterm neonates exposed to iodine. J Perinat Med 2017;45(1):135–43.
28. Thaker VV, Leung AM, Braverman LE, et al. Iodine-induced hypothyroidism in full-term infants with congenital heart disease: more common than currently appreciated? J Clin Endocrinol Metab 2014;99(10):3521–6.
29. Chung HR, Shin CH, Yang SW, et al. Subclinical hypothyroidism in Korean preterm infants associated with high levels of iodine in breast milk. J Clin Endocrinol Metab 2009;94(11):4444–7.
30. Connelly KJ, Boston BA, Pearce EN, et al. Congenital hypothyroidism caused by excess prenatal maternal iodine ingestion. J Pediatr 2012;161(4):760–2.
31. Hanna CE, Krainz PL, Skeels MR, et al. Detection of congenital hypopituitary hypothyroidism: ten-year experience in the Northwest Regional Screening Program. J Pediatr 1986;109(6):959–64.
32. Lanting CI, van Tijn DA, Loeber JG, et al. Clinical effectiveness and cost-effectiveness of the use of the thyroxine/thyroxine-binding globulin ratio to detect congenital hypothyroidism of thyroidal and central origin in a neonatal screening program. Pediatrics 2005;116(1):168–73.
33. van Tijn DA, de Vijlder JJ, Verbeeten B Jr, et al. Neonatal detection of congenital hypothyroidism of central origin. J Clin Endocrinol Metab 2005;90(6):3350–9.
34. Schoenmakers N, Alatzoglou KS, Chatterjee VK, et al. Recent advances in central congenital hypothyroidism. J Endocrinol 2015;227(3):R51–71.
35. Sun Y, Bak B, Schoenmakers N, et al. Loss-of-function mutations in IGSF1 cause an X-linked syndrome of central hypothyroidism and testicular enlargement. Nat Genet 2012;44(12):1375–81.
36. Garcia M, Barrio R, Garcia-Lavandeira M, et al. The syndrome of central hypothyroidism and macroorchidism: IGSF1 controls TRHR and FSHB expression by differential modulation of pituitary TGFbeta and Activin pathways. Sci Rep 2017;7:42937.
37. Turgeon MO, Silander TL, Doycheva D, et al. TRH action is impaired in pituitaries of male IGSF1-deficient mice. Endocrinology 2017;158(4):815–30.
38. Collu R, Tang J, Castagne J, et al. A novel mechanism for isolated central hypothyroidism: inactivating mutations in the thyrotropin-releasing hormone receptor gene. J Clin Endocrinol Metab 1997;82(5):1561–5.
39. Nicholas AK, Jaleel S, Lyons G, et al. Molecular spectrum of TSHbeta subunit gene defects in central hypothyroidism in the UK and Ireland. Clin Endocrinol (Oxf) 2017;86(3):410–8.
40. Heinen CA, Losekoot M, Sun Y, et al. Mutations in TBL1X are associated with central hypothyroidism. J Clin Endocrinol Metab 2016;101(12):4564–73.
41. Lichtenberger-Geslin L, Dos Santos S, Hassani Y, et al. Factors associated with hearing impairment in patients with congenital hypothyroidism treated since the neonatal period: a national population-based study. J Clin Endocrinol Metab 2013;98(9):3644–52.
42. Dimitri P, Habeb AM, Gurbuz F, et al. Expanding the clinical spectrum associated with GLIS3 mutations. J Clin Endocrinol Metab 2015;100(10):E1362–9.
43. Ford G, LaFranchi SH. Screening for congenital hypothyroidism: a worldwide view of strategies. Best Pract Res Clin Endocrinol Metab 2014;28(2):175–87.
44. Nebesio TD, McKenna MP, Nabhan ZM, et al. Newborn screening results in children with central hypothyroidism. J Pediatr 2010;156(6):990–3.
45. Leger J, Olivieri A, Donaldson M, et al. European Society for Paediatric Endocrinology consensus guidelines on screening, diagnosis, and management of congenital hypothyroidism. Horm Res Paediatr 2014;81(2):80–103.

46. Fisher DA, Odell WD. Acute release of thyrotropin in the newborn. J Clin Invest 1969;48(9):1670–7.
47. LaFranchi SH, Hanna CE, Krainz PL, et al. Screening for congenital hypothyroidism with specimen collection at two time periods: results of the Northwest Regional Screening Program. Pediatrics 1985;76(5):734–40.
48. Larson C, Hermos R, Delaney A, et al. Risk factors associated with delayed thyrotropin elevations in congenital hypothyroidism. J Pediatr 2003;143(5):587–91.
49. Woo HC, Lizarda A, Tucker R, et al. Congenital hypothyroidism with a delayed thyroid-stimulating hormone elevation in very premature infants: incidence and growth and developmental outcomes. J Pediatr 2011;158(4):538–42.
50. Slaughter JL, Meinzen-Derr J, Rose SR, et al. The effects of gestational age and birth weight on false-positive newborn-screening rates. Pediatrics 2010;126(5): 910–6.
51. Ford GA, Denniston S, Sesser D, et al. Transient versus permanent congenital hypothyroidism after the age of 3 years in infants detected on the first versus second newborn screening test in Oregon, USA. Horm Res Paediatr 2016;86(3): 169–77.
52. Williams FL, Simpson J, Delahunty C, et al. Developmental trends in cord and postpartum serum thyroid hormones in preterm infants. J Clin Endocrinol Metab 2004;89(11):5314–20.
53. Trumpff C, De Schepper J, Vanderfaeillie J, et al. Thyroid-stimulating hormone (TSH) concentration at birth in Belgian neonates and cognitive development at preschool age. Nutrients 2015;7(11):9018–32.
54. Trumpff C, De Schepper J, Vanderfaeillie J, et al. Neonatal thyroid-stimulating hormone concentration and psychomotor development at preschool age. Arch Dis Child 2016;101(12):1100–6.
55. Lain SJ, Bentley JP, Wiley V, et al. Association between borderline neonatal thyroid-stimulating hormone concentrations and educational and developmental outcomes: a population-based record-linkage study. Lancet Diabetes Endocrinol 2016;4(9):756–65.
56. Rabbiosi S, Vigone MC, Cortinovis F, et al. Congenital hypothyroidism with eutopic thyroid gland: analysis of clinical and biochemical features at diagnosis and after re-evaluation. J Clin Endocrinol Metab 2013;98(4):1395–402.
57. Jin HY, Heo SH, Kim YM, et al. High frequency of DUOX2 mutations in transient or permanent congenital hypothyroidism with eutopic thyroid glands. Horm Res Paediatr 2014;82(4):252–60.
58. Castanet M, Goischke A, Leger J, et al. Natural history and management of congenital hypothyroidism with in situ thyroid gland. Horm Res Paediatr 2015; 83(2):102–10.
59. La Gamma EF, Paneth N. Clinical importance of hypothyroxinemia in the preterm infant and a discussion of treatment concerns. Curr Opin Pediatr 2012;24(2): 172–80.
60. Rose SR, Brown RS, Foley T, et al. Update of newborn screening and therapy for congenital hypothyroidism. Pediatrics 2006;117(6):2290–303.
61. Bongers-Schokking JJ, Koot HM, Wiersma D, et al. Influence of timing and dose of thyroid hormone replacement on development in infants with congenital hypothyroidism. J Pediatr 2000;136(3):292–7.
62. Selva KA, Harper A, Downs A, et al. Neurodevelopmental outcomes in congenital hypothyroidism: comparison of initial T4 dose and time to reach target T4 and TSH. J Pediatr 2005;147(6):775–80.

63. Chorazy PA, Himelhoch S, Hopwood NJ, et al. Persistent hypothyroidism in an infant receiving a soy formula: case report and review of the literature. Pediatrics 1995;96(1 Pt 1):148–50.
64. Conrad SC, Chiu H, Silverman BL. Soy formula complicates management of congenital hypothyroidism. Arch Dis Child 2004;89(1):37–40.
65. Jonklaas J, Bianco AC, Bauer AJ, et al. Guidelines for the treatment of hypothyroidism: prepared by the American Thyroid Association task force on thyroid hormone replacement. Thyroid 2014;24(12):1670–751.
66. New England Congenital Hypothyroidism Collaborative. Correlation of cognitive test scores and adequacy of treatment in adolescents with congenital hypothyroidism. New England Congenital Hypothyroidism Collaborative. J Pediatr 1994;124(3):383–7.
67. Heyerdahl S, Kase BF. Significance of elevated serum thyrotropin during treatment of congenital hypothyroidism. Acta Paediatr 1995;84(6):634–8.
68. Leger J, Larroque B, Norton J, Association Française pour le Dépistage et la Prévetion des Handicaps de l'Enfant. Influence of severity of congenital hypothyroidism and adequacy of treatment on school achievement in young adolescents: a population-based cohort study. Acta Paediatr 2001;90(11):1249–56.
69. Oerbeck B, Sundet K, Kase BF, et al. Congenital hypothyroidism: influence of disease severity and L-thyroxine treatment on intellectual, motor, and school-associated outcomes in young adults. Pediatrics 2003;112(4):923–30.
70. Alvarez M, Iglesias Fernandez C, Rodriguez Sanchez A, et al. Episodes of overtreatment during the first six months in children with congenital hypothyroidism and their relationships with sustained attention and inhibitory control at school age. Horm Res Paediatr 2010;74(2):114–20.
71. Bongers-Schokking JJ, Resing WC, de Rijke YB, et al. Cognitive development in congenital hypothyroidism: is overtreatment a greater threat than undertreatment? J Clin Endocrinol Metab 2013;98(11):4499–506.
72. Vaidyanathan P, Pathak M, Kaplowitz PB. In congenital hypothyroidism, an initial L-thyroxine dose of 10-12 mug/kg/day is sufficient and sometimes excessive based on thyroid tests 1 month later. J Pediatr Endocrinol Metab 2012;25(9–10):849–52.
73. Elmlinger MW, Kuhnel W, Lambrecht HG, et al. Reference intervals from birth to adulthood for serum thyroxine (T4), triiodothyronine (T3), free T3, free T4, thyroxine binding globulin (TBG) and thyrotropin (TSH). Clin Chem Lab Med 2001;39(10):973–9.
74. Chaler EA, Fiorenzano R, Chilelli C, et al. Age-specific thyroid hormone and thyrotropin reference intervals for a pediatric and adolescent population. Clin Chem Lab Med 2012;50(5):885–90.
75. Bailey D, Colantonio D, Kyriakopoulou L, et al. Marked biological variance in endocrine and biochemical markers in childhood: establishment of pediatric reference intervals using healthy community children from the CALIPER cohort. Clin Chem 2013;59(9):1393–405.
76. Fisher DA, Schoen EJ, La Franchi S, et al. The hypothalamic-pituitary-thyroid negative feedback control axis in children with treated congenital hypothyroidism. J Clin Endocrinol Metab 2000;85(8):2722–7.
77. Simoneau-Roy J, Marti S, Deal C, et al. Cognition and behavior at school entry in children with congenital hypothyroidism treated early with high-dose levothyroxine. J Pediatr 2004;144(6):747–52.
78. Bongers-Schokking JJ, de Muinck Keizer-Schrama SM. Influence of timing and dose of thyroid hormone replacement on mental, psychomotor, and behavioral

development in children with congenital hypothyroidism. J Pediatr 2005;147(6): 768–74.

79. Leger J. Congenital hypothyroidism: a clinical update of long-term outcome in young adults. Eur J Endocrinol 2015;172(2):R67–77.

Thyroid Function in the Neonatal Intensive Care Unit

Monika Chaudhari, MD[a], Jonathan L. Slaughter, MD, MPH[b],*

KEYWORDS

- Congenital hypothyroidism • Neonatal intensive care unit • Preterm infants
- Thyroid screening • Thyroid function testing • Thyroid testing artifacts

KEY POINTS

- Neonatal illness and prematurity may necessitate additional thyroid function screening to ensure early detection and treatment of hypothyroidism, and may alter the results and interpretation of thyroid function tests.
- Preterm infants are prone to transient hypothyroidism with delayed thyroid stimulating hormone (TSH) rise because of immaturity of the hypothalamic-pituitary-thyroid axis at birth.
- Transiently low total thyroxine (T4) and triiodothyronine (T3) levels are common during periods of neonatal illness in term and preterm infants.

INTRODUCTION

The neonatal intensive care unit (NICU) presents unique challenges to routine universal newborn thyroid screening for early detection and treatment of congenital hypothyroidism, and the interpretation of collected thyroid function tests (TFTs).[1] Preterm infants are born before hypothalamic-pituitary-thyroid axis maturation and are prone to hypothyroidism with delayed thyroid-stimulating hormone (TSH) rise and transient hypothyroidism.[2,3] In addition, illness affects the interpretation of TFTs of preterm and term sick infants.[4,5]

This article reviews normal fetal and neonatal hypothalamic-pituitary-thyroid axis development, indications for and timing of thyroid hormone testing in the NICU, medication artifacts and conditions that may affect thyroid test results, thyroid test interpretation in the NICU, evidence for and against providing thyroid hormone to NICU

Disclosure Statement: The authors have no financial relationships to disclose.
[a] Department of Pediatrics, Division of Endocrinology, Nationwide Children's Hospital, The Ohio State University, 700 Children's Crossroad, Columbus, OH 43205, USA; [b] Department of Pediatrics, Division of Neonatology, Center for Perinatal Research, Nationwide Children's Hospital, The Ohio State University, Research 3 Building, 575 Children's Crossroad, Columbus, OH 43215, USA
* Corresponding author.
E-mail address: Jonathan.Slaughter@nationwidechildrens.org

Clin Perinatol 45 (2018) 19–30
https://doi.org/10.1016/j.clp.2017.10.005
0095-5108/18/© 2017 Elsevier Inc. All rights reserved.

patients who have borderline TFT, and follow-up retesting of NICU infants with hypothyroidism, to differentiate transient from permanent hypothyroidism.

NORMAL IN UTERO AND POSTNATAL HYPOTHALAMIC-PITUITARY AXIS DEVELOPMENT

During the first trimester, the fetus must derive all of its thyroid hormone supply from the mother.[6] Maternal unbound thyroxine (free T4) levels increase in early pregnancy when placental human chorionic gonadotrophin, structurally similar to TSH, exhibits a weak TSH-like effect.[7] Free T4 remains elevated throughout pregnancy and is actively transported across the placenta via thyroid hormone transporters.[8,9] Although total thyroxine (T4) levels in the fetal compartments are 1/100th of maternal levels, the unbound and active fraction, free T4, is elevated relative to adults.[8,10] Iodine is also actively transported across the placenta.[11] Within the brain, type 2 and type 3 deiodinases locally convert T4 to T3, which is critical to embryonic neural cell development.[6,12]

The thyroid is the earliest endocrine structure to develop. The thyroid placode, an enlargement of the embryonic endoderm, is noted by embryonic day 22.[13] The developing thyroid begins to collect and store iodine by 10 to 12 weeks.[14] Thyroid follicles have developed by the time the fetal thyroid begins to secrete hormones into the circulation at approximately 16 weeks.[6,11] The parafollicular cells (C-cells), the neuroendocrine cells in the thyroid that produce calcitonin, develop separately. These cells differentiate from the ectoderm and move into the interfollicular connective tissue during thyroid gland development.[15] The hypothalamus develops in the first and second trimesters and it begins to take on an adult-like appearance between 24 and 33 weeks.[16,17]

T4 and free T4 serum concentrations continue to rise until they reach adult levels by 36-weeks' gestation.[18] Thyroxine-binding globulin, the primary carrier of bound T4 in the bloodstream, also rises during the second half of pregnancy.[19] However, serum concentrations of T3 and free T3 remain low throughout fetal development before a late surge prior to term.[18]

At birth, TSH, T3, and free T4 levels rapidly rise within the first postnatal half-hour.[18] However, this rise is attenuated in preterm infants because of hypothalamic-pituitary-thyroid axis immaturity. The degree of rise correlates inversely with gestational age and in the most extremely preterm infants, thyroid hormone levels decrease in the hours following birth.[20]

APPROPRIATE INDICATIONS FOR AND APPROPRIATE TIMING OF THYROID HORMONE TESTING

Congenital hypothyroidism is the most common disorder that is screened for on universal newborn metabolic screens. All infants hospitalized within the NICU should receive an initial thyroid screening test within several days of birth.[19,21] Usually this is done as part of government-mandated and -sponsored universal newborn metabolic screening. The test should be collected after 24-hours postnatal age, whenever possible, which reduces the false-positive rate especially in preterm NICU patients.[21,22] If government-sponsored metabolic screens must be collected before 24-hours because of blood transfusions that would interfere with screening results, it is important to always repeat a second screen after 24-hours postnatal age.

It must be remembered that infants may develop congenital hypothyroidism even if the initial screen within the first several days after birth had normal TSH and T4.

NICU patients, including preterm infants and acutely ill infants, are at high risk for hypothyroidism with delayed TSH rise.[3] Compared with more mature infants, the prevalence of congenital hypothyroidism is higher in very low birth weight (VLBW) (<1500 g) neonates.[2,4,23] VLBW infants reportedly have a 14-fold higher incidence of transient hypothyroidism compared with infants that are greater than 1500 g at birth, although levels of permanent hypothyroidism are similar in preterm and term infants.[4,24,25] Most VLBW newborns with congenital hypothyroidism initially have a normal government newborn screening test and subsequently have a delayed TSH elevation.[4,24–26]

The 2014 European Society for Pediatric Endocrinology Consensus Guidelines on Screening, Diagnosis, and Management of Congenital Hypothyroidism[5] state that a second screening may be required for preterm neonates born at a gestation less than 37 weeks, for infants with a birthweight less than 1500 g, for ill and pre-term neonates admitted to the NICU, if the initial specimen collection was collected in the first 24 hours postnatal, or if there are multiple births which may have permitted mixing of blood secondary to twin-twin transfusion. The guidelines recommend that a repeat specimen should be collected at 2-weeks postnatal age or 2 weeks after the first screen was obtained.[5] These factors have led most newborn screening programs to recommend rescreening of preterm infants. However, there are no standardized guidelines currently in place and the indications and timing for rescreening remain debatable. Some recommend rescreening at 2 weeks[1]; others at 4 weeks[27] and 6 weeks.[2] Within the United States, some states recommend an additional government newborn screen via dried blood spot, whereas others recommend obtaining in-house serum TFT as a repeat screen. In the absence of a universal repeat screening protocol for preterm infants, it is critical that clinicians obtain a serum TSH and free T4 whenever there is a clinical concern for potential thyroid disorder.[1]

ARTIFACTS AND CONDITIONS THAT MAY AFFECT THYROID FUNCTION TEST INTERPRETATION

A variety of issues can affect the TFTs. The most common are associated with prematurity, illness, medications, and maternal thyroid disease.

Iodine

Preterm infants born at less than 32 weeks are vulnerable to thyroid dysfunction because of the effects of iodine.[28] The normal human defense mechanism against iodine overload, called the Wolff-Chaikoff effect, prevents overproduction of thyroid hormone once serum iodine reaches a critical level by stopping the uptake of iodine and iodination of tyrosine.[28] However, Wolff-Chaikoff is not typically mature until 36 to 40 weeks' gestation. Immaturity of the thyroid gland, increased permeability of the skin, and decreased renal clearance of iodine in preterm infants also contribute to iodine-associated thyroid dysfunction.[28–30] Iodine overload can be caused by iodinated disinfectants, iodinated contrast media, and high maternal iodine concentrations (prenatally through skin disinfection with povidone iodine used in C-section, vaginal douching, epidural/spinal anesthesia, or postnatally through breast milk).[28,31] If iodine overload is suspected, urinary iodine levels should be measured and the TFTs closely monitored. In a recent systematic review, the incidence of transient hypothyroidism/hyperthyrotropinemia in iodine-exposed infants ranged from 12% to 33%[28,29] depending on the laboratory values used to classify hypothyroidism. Some defined hypothyroidism as a TSH greater than 20 mIU/L and some as TSH greater than

30 mIU/L,[28] with a definition of hyperthyrotropinemia for TSH greater than or equal to 10 but less than or equal to 20 mIU/L.[28]

Nonthyroidal Illness

Nonthyroidal illness (NTI), otherwise also known as sick euthyroid syndrome, can cause changes in serum levels of thyroidal hormones in the absence of classical thyroidal disease. The classic picture seen in NTI is low serum total T3, normal to low total T4, elevated reverse T3, and normal TSH levels. These alterations are believed to be adaptive for the individual and the severity of illness has been correlated with the magnitude of changes observed.[32] In newborn infants, a low T3 is the most frequent change that is seen and an elevation of reverse T3 is not always observed. The low levels of T3 are thought to be an adaptive response to stress to save energy, reduce the metabolic rate, and protect the body from hypercatabolism caused by illness.[33–35] The lower the total T3 value, the poorer the prognosis for infant survival and the more metabolically adaptive it may be for the infant to have the low T3 level. When clinical recovery occurs, a rise in TSH should be followed by an increase in serum T3.[32] Illness severity can also have an impact. Sick premature infants have an attenuated hypothalamic-pituitary-thyroid axis response secondary to immaturity. With critical illness, they are exposed to a variety of agents known to affect TFT. In cases of neonatal sepsis or septic shock, thyroid hormone levels may have a possible prognostic value but further studies need to be completed. Interleukin-6 and other inflammatory cytokines, components of the acute phase response during illness, have been implicated in the pathogenesis of NTI. Low levels of total T3 and T4 are associated with illnesses and adverse outcomes including respiratory distress syndrome, sepsis, and mortality.[36]

Medications

Several medications are known to affect TFT results. Dopamine is an adrenergic neurotransmitter that inhibits TSH secretion by means of adenylyl cyclase. This blockage may be caused by gene expression inhibition for the B subunit of TSH leading to an inhibition of nocturnal TSH peak amplitude.[34] Dopamine also suppresses T4 secretion. Once dopamine is discontinued, an immediate increase in T4 levels can occur.[37,38]

Steroid or glucocorticoid use can lead to a reduction in T3 and an elevation of reverse T3 approximately 12 hours after starting the medication.[34] Steroid use can also reduce the TSH response and peripheral conversion of T4 to T3.[37] Arai and colleagues[37] demonstrated that infants undergoing steroid exposure at 2 weeks of age had significantly lower TSH levels than those without steroid exposure.

Metoclopramide, a dopamine receptor antagonist, is used to prompt gastric emptying in neonates with gastrointestinal dysmotility issues and can induce a significant TSH release resulting in transient thyroid dysfunction.[39]

Aminophylline, caffeine, and the active metabolite theophylline are used as respiratory stimulants for neonatal apnea. These medications can increase the expression of TSH and thyroglobulin, which then can result in thyroid dysfunction.[39]

Heparin used intravenously or subcutaneously, even in very small doses, such as to keep a cannula patent, can cause competition for the thyroid hormone binding sites on thyroid binding globulin and artifactually increase the serum free thyroid hormone levels. Therefore it is best to avoid measuring the free T4 during this time but if clinically indicated, then obtain the blood sample greater than 10 hours after the last injection of heparin and analyze the sample without delay. If displacement is suspected, measure total T4 along with TSH and thyroid binding globulin to help confirm the patient's thyroid status.[40–42]

Maternal Factors

Maternal TSH receptor blocking antibodies and maternal thyroid medications can also affect the TFTs in the neonate leading to a higher likelihood of having transient disease. Therefore, it is important to try to identify mothers with severe autoimmune thyroid disease so that the neonate's thyroid function can be closely monitored.[43,44] Maternal iodine deficiency and maternal iodine excess (either through nutritional supplements, iodine-rich seaweed, kelp, brassica vegetables) can also cause inadequate thyroid hormone levels.[30,45] Although less common in industrialized nations, iodine deficiency is the most common cause of congenital hypothyroidism worldwide.[5]

INTERPRETATION OF TESTS OF THYROID FUNCTION

The interpretation of TFTs in sick and preterm infants is complex. Although there are numerous reasons for abnormal TFT results in preterm neonates, the most common is immaturity of the hypothalamic-pituitary-thyroid axis. The feedback loop of the hypothalamic-pituitary-thyroid axis is not fully developed, which results in delayed TSH rise in response to serum levels of thyroid hormones. Other common reasons for abnormal screening results in hospitalized neonates, apart from true permanent congenital hypothyroidism, include exposure to certain, commonly used drugs in the neonatal period, inability to regulate iodine balance, and postnatal illnesses.[2]

TSH elevation is common in preterm infants within the first postnatal month when they are critically ill and have possible exposure to various medications. This often makes it unclear if initial TSH elevations are caused by permanent hypothyroidism, persistent hyperthyrotropinemia (elevated TSH with normal T4), or transient hypothyroidism.[2,4,23,25] As preterm infants recover from hypothyroxinemia (low free T4 level with normal TSH level), some have mild transient serum TSH level elevation before reaching a new equilibrium. When followed over time, the TSH returns to normal in most and is considered a normal response to the physiologic hypothyroxinemia seen in healthy preterm infants.[4] Some preterm infants have greater and more persistent delayed TSH elevation. This is either transient or permanent. There do not seem to be any clinical or laboratory characteristics that reliably predict whether the hypothyroidism will be transient or permanent. Woo and colleagues[4] analyzed LBW infants with initial low screening T4 and normal TSH. On repeat screenings, 85% had moderate TSH elevation that normalized spontaneously without treatment at an average of 42 days. The other 15% with higher TSH values were started on treatment.[4]

There are currently no universal standards in place for values used to signify a positive congenital hypothyroidism result based on TSH. When newborn screening was initiated, a blood spot TSH value of 30 mIU/L was the cutoff. Then in the 1990s, the cutoff point was lowered to 20 mIU/L. Following documented cases of congenital hypothyroidism that were missed, studies were performed using a TSH threshold of 10 mIU/L.[46] Mengreli and colleagues[46] found that 65% of preterm infants with permanent congenital hypothyroidism were detected using a TSH cutoff value of greater than 10 mIU/L on the first newborn screen. However, the call-back rate for positive screens with this lower TSH cutoff value was increased 10-fold from baseline to 1.2%.[46]

Some have suggested that if a lower TSH threshold were used, a second TSH screen might not be necessary.[47]

The mean T4 is lower in VLBW infants relative to infants weighing greater than 1500 g. This is most likely secondary to low thyroid binding globulin levels and increased incidence of NTI (sick euthyroid syndrome).[4] Gestational age and birth weight specific reference ranges have been published to aid clinicians in their interpretation of TFT in hospitalized preterm infants. Sun and colleagues[24] established reference intervals for VLBW infants (mean gestational age, 27.9 weeks; mean birthweight, 992 g) at 3 to 6 weeks of age: the normal free T4 range is 0.85 to 1.7 ng/dL and TSH range is 1.14 to 11.04 mIU/L.

EVIDENCE FOR AND AGAINST PROVIDING THYROID HORMONE TO NEONATAL INTENSIVE CARE UNIT PATIENTS WHO HAVE BORDERLINE THYROID FUNCTION TESTS

It is well known that thyroid hormones are required for normal human brain development and that replacement of thyroid deficiency in full-term infants is indicated as early as possible to prevent neurodevelopmental problems.[1] However, the treatment indications and guidelines for hospitalized infants with transient or mild thyroid abnormalities continue to be debated.

Universal Levothyroxine Supplementation for Very Low Birth Weight Preterm Infants

Because transient hypothyroidism is common in preterm infants due to hypothalamic-pituitary-thyroid axis immaturity, it was hypothesized that routinely supplementing all VLBW preterm infants with levothyroxine (L-T4) would improve neurodevelopment. However, multiple randomized trials showed no benefit. Van Wassenaer and coinvestigators[48] found universal thyroxine supplementation to infants born at less than 30 weeks' gestation had no effect on 24-month neurodevelopmental outcomes. A multicenter, double-blind randomized placebo-controlled trial by Ng and colleagues[49] that assessed the effects of L-T4 supplementation for all less than 28 weeks' gestation infants, found no apparent effect on brain size and growth at 36 weeks' postmenstrual age. Van Wassernaer-Leemhuis and colleagues[50] performed a multicenter, phase 1 clinical trial of differing doses of thyroid hormone supplementation for infants born at less than 28 week's gestation and assessed 3-year neurodevelopmental outcomes. There were no differences in cognitive, motor, and neurologic development in the treated versus the nontreated groups, nor were there adverse outcomes in the treated group.

Although rare, L-T4 supplementation has been associated with adverse effects. Kawai and colleagues[51] found in a nationwide surveillance study that late-onset circulatory collapse was reported in 0.5% of infants that received L-T4. It was hypothesized that L-T4 may have increased the relative adrenal insufficiency of prematurity and thus the risk of late-onset circulatory collapse in VLBW infants. If L-T4 is used in VLBW infants, close monitoring of blood pressure and adrenal function should occur.[51]

Transient Hypothyroidism

Transient hypothyroxinemia (low free T4 level with normal TSH) is common in preterm neonates and has been associated with later neurodevelopmental deficiency.[52,53] However, the exact serum levels of free T4 needed to achieve optimal brain maturation have not been quantified and there is no universal consensus on an age or free T4 level cutoff at which treatment should be mandatory.[54] It is possible that low thyroid

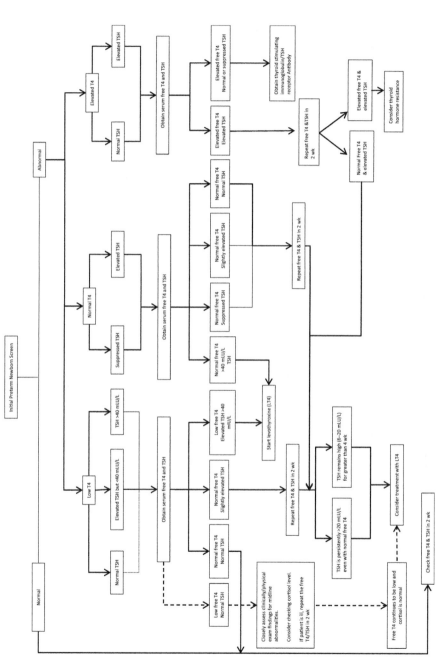

Fig. 1. Flowchart to assist in decision making for rescreening and treating hypothyroidism in preterm infants.

hormone levels are a normal physiologic attempt to protect the sick infant by reducing the metabolic rate during a time of illness.[37]

Transient congenital hypothyroidism with delayed TSH rise is also common in preterm infants.[1] The benefit of treating premature infants with transient TSH elevations with L-T4 is unclear. Some researchers recommend that neonates, even with transiently elevated TSH values (>50 mIU/L), should be promptly treated with L-T4 because of intellectual disability risk.[2] Woo and colleagues[4] found that at 18-month follow-up, VLBW infants with a history of congenital hypothyroidism with delayed TSH elevation had similar growth and neurodevelopment as compared with matched control subjects without hypothyroidism. However, they noted significantly more head circumferences measuring less than 10th percentile in infants with hypothyroidism with delayed TSH elevation.[4]

Uchiyama and colleagues[55] performed an unmasked, multicenter randomized clinical trial of L-T4 supplementation in VLBW infants with transient hypothyroxinemia of prematurity. Infants with TSH less than 10 mIU/L and free T4 less than 0.8 ng/L were randomized to L-T4 supplementation or placebo between 2 and 4 weeks of age. L-T4 treatment did not affect growth or neurodevelopmental outcome at 18 months and 3 month of age.[55,56]

Fig. 1 presents a flowchart to assist in decision making for rescreening and treating hypothyroidism in preterm infants. Given the complexity of TFT evaluation in sick and preterm neonates, we recommend consultation with a pediatric endocrinologist when deciding when to begin treatment and for planning follow-up. Regardless of initial treatment decision, close monitoring of patients with borderline elevated TSH values is important because persistent or permanent hypothyroidism is noted in a subset of infants.[2]

WHEN TO RETEST TO ASSESS PERMANENCY OF HYPOTHYROIDISM

The American Academy of Pediatrics[1] recommends assessing the permanency of congenital hypothyroidism in children treated with L-T4 if the initial TSH was less than 50 mIU/L without an increase in TSH during therapy following the newborn period. Assessment for permanent congenital hypothyroidism should be performed after 3 years of age, by either a trial off therapy for 30 days or a 50% reduction in the dose of L-T4 for 30 days. Subsequent repeat TFTs should be collected to assess the effects. If the TFTs were normal after the 50% L-T4 dose reduction, then medication should be discontinued for 30 days and the TFTs repeated. If the TSH is elevated off of therapy, this would be compatible with hypothyroidism.

SUMMARY

Compared with healthy term newborns, infants hospitalized within NICUs are more likely to have abnormal TFTs because of illness and prematurity. Because of an immature hypothalamic-pituitary-thyroid axis, preterm infants may present with congenital hypothyroidism with a delayed TSH rise that is undetected on initial postnatal screening tests. Therefore, repeat screening several weeks after birth is recommended.[5] Congenital hypothyroidism in NICU patients may be transient, and consultation with a pediatric endocrinologist is recommended when deciding when to begin treatment. Regardless of initial treatment decisions, it is important to closely follow serum TSH and free T4 levels to exclude the possibility of permanent hypothyroidism.

Best Practices

What is the current practice?

Newborn screening for congenital hypothyroidism
All newborns including those hospitalized in NICUs should receive TSH and T4 based screening for congenital hypothyroidism in the first several days after birth. Screens should be collected after 24-hours postnatal age unless earlier screen collection is necessitated by blood transfusion. Screens collected before 24 hours should be repeated, because the results have high likelihood of being false positive.

What changes in current practice are likely to improve outcomes?

- Thyroid screening tests should be repeated in sick and preterm NICU patients at several weeks postnatal age to evaluate for congenital hypothyroidism with delayed TSH rise.

- It is important to closely follow abnormal serum TSH and free T4 levels in 2-week intervals, to assess for permanent hypothyroidism.

- If the TSH is greater than 40 mIU/L, start levothyroxine therapy (10–15 μg/kg orally daily; intravenous dose is ~50% of oral dose)

- If the TSH is elevated but less than 40 mIU/L, repeat the free T4 and TSH levels.

- If the TSH is persistently elevated at 4-weeks postnatal age, consider levothyroxine therapy (10–15 μg/kg orally daily; intravenous dose is ~50% of oral dose)

- Once levothyroxine therapy is initiated, repeat the free T4 and TSH in 4 weeks to assess adequacy of the dose.

- Consider a trial off therapy at 3 years of age in those individuals who had a normal free T4 with an elevated TSH, to determine whether lifelong therapy is needed.

Is there a clinical algorithm?

The most common clinical recommendations for neonatal screening, diagnosis, and treatment of congenital hypothyroidism are those of the American Academy of Pediatrics and the European Society for Paediatric Endocrinology.

Data from Rose SR, Brown RS, Foley T, et al. Update of newborn screening and therapy for congenital hypothyroidism. Pediatrics 2006;117(6):2290–303; and Leger J, Olivieri A, Donaldson M, et al. European Society for Paediatric Endocrinology consensus guidelines on screening, diagnosis, and management of congenital hypothyroidism. J Clin Endocrinol Metab 2014;99(2):363–84.

REFERENCES

1. American Academy of Pediatrics, Rose SR, Section on Endocrinology and Committee on Genetics, American Thyroid Association, et al. Update of newborn screening and therapy for congenital hypothyroidism. Pediatrics 2006;117(6): 2290–303.

2. Vigone MC, Caiulo S, Di Frenna M, et al. Evolution of thyroid function in preterm infants detected by screening for congenital hypothyroidism. J Pediatr 2014; 164(6):1296–302.

3. LaFranchi SH. Newborn screening strategies for congenital hypothyroidism: an update. J Inherit Metab Dis 2010;33(Suppl 2):S225–33.

4. Woo HC, Lizarda A, Tucker R, et al. Congenital hypothyroidism with a delayed thyroid-stimulating hormone elevation in very premature infants: incidence and growth and developmental outcomes. J Pediatr 2011;158(4): 538–42.

5. Leger J, Olivieri A, Donaldson M, et al. European Society for Paediatric Endocrinology consensus guidelines on screening, diagnosis, and management of congenital hypothyroidism. J Clin Endocrinol Metab 2014;99(2):363–84.

6. Obregon MJ, Calvo RM, Del Rey FE, et al. Ontogenesis of thyroid function and interactions with maternal function. Endocr Dev 2007;10:86–98.

7. Pekonen F, Alfthan H, Stenman UH, et al. Human chorionic gonadotropin (hCG) and thyroid function in early human pregnancy: circadian variation and evidence for intrinsic thyrotropic activity of hCG. J Clin Endocrinol Metab 1988;66(4):853–6.

8. Calvo RM, Jauniaux E, Gulbis B, et al. Fetal tissues are exposed to biologically relevant free thyroxine concentrations during early phases of development. J Clin Endocrinol Metab 2002;87(4):1768–77.

9. Loubiere LS, Vasilopoulou E, Glazier JD, et al. Expression and function of thyroid hormone transporters in the microvillous plasma membrane of human term placental syncytiotrophoblast. Endocrinology 2012;153(12):6126–35.

10. Contempre B, Jauniaux E, Calvo R, et al. Detection of thyroid hormones in human embryonic cavities during the first trimester of pregnancy. J Clin Endocrinol Metab 1993;77(6):1719–22.

11. Forhead AJ, Fowden AL. Thyroid hormones in fetal growth and prepartum maturation. J Endocrinol 2014;221(3):R87–103.

12. Kester MH, Martinez de Mena R, Obregon MJ, et al. Iodothyronine levels in the human developing brain: major regulatory roles of iodothyronine deiodinases in different areas. J Clin Endocrinol Metab 2004;89(7):3117–28.

13. De Felice M, Di Lauro R. Minireview: intrinsic and extrinsic factors in thyroid gland development: an update. Endocrinology 2011;152(8):2948–56.

14. Burrow GN, Fisher DA, Larsen PR. Maternal and fetal thyroid function. N Engl J Med 1994;331(16):1072–8.

15. Stathatos N. Thyroid physiology. Med Clin North Am 2012;96(2):165–73.

16. Koutcherov Y, Mai JK, Ashwell KW, et al. Organization of human hypothalamus in fetal development. J Comp Neurol 2002;446(4):301–24.

17. Friesema EC, Visser TJ, Borgers AJ, et al. Thyroid hormone transporters and deiodinases in the developing human hypothalamus. Eur J Endocrinol 2012;167(3):379–86.

18. Thorpe-Beeston JG, Nicolaides KH, Felton CV, et al. Maturation of the secretion of thyroid hormone and thyroid-stimulating hormone in the fetus. N Engl J Med 1991;324(8):532–6.

19. Rapaport R, Rose SR, Freemark M. Hypothyroxinemia in the preterm infant: the benefits and risks of thyroxine treatment. J Pediatr 2001;139(2):182–8.

20. Murphy N, Hume R, van Toor H, et al. The hypothalamic-pituitary-thyroid axis in preterm infants; changes in the first 24 hours of postnatal life. J Clin Endocrinol Metab 2004;89(6):2824–31.

21. Slaughter JL, Meinzen-Derr J, Rose SR, et al. The effects of gestational age and birth weight on false-positive newborn-screening rates. Pediatrics 2010;126(5):910–6.

22. Lott JA, Sardovia-Iyer M, Speakman KS, et al. Age-dependent cutoff values in screening newborns for hypothyroidism. Clin Biochem 2004;37(9):791–7.

23. Corbetta C, Weber G, Cortinovis F, et al. A 7-year experience with low blood TSH cutoff levels for neonatal screening reveals an unsuspected frequency of congenital hypothyroidism (CH). Clin Endocrinol 2009;71(5):739–45.

24. Sun X, Lemyre B, Nan X, et al. Free thyroxine and thyroid-stimulating hormone reference intervals in very low birth weight infants at 3-6 weeks of life with the Beckman Coulter Unicel Dxl 800. Clin Biochem 2014;47(1–2):16–8.

25. Larson C, Hermos R, Delaney A, et al. Risk factors associated with delayed thyrotropin elevations in congenital hypothyroidism. J Pediatr 2003;143(5):587–91.
26. Silva SA, Chagas AJ, Goulart EM, et al. Screening for congenital hypothyroidism in extreme premature and/or very low birth weight newborns: the importance of a specific protocol. J Pediatr Endocrinol Metab 2010;23(1–2):45–52.
27. Bijarnia S, Wilcken B, Wiley VC. Newborn screening for congenital hypothyroidism in very-low-birth-weight babies: the need for a second test. J Inherit Metab Dis 2011;34(3):827–33.
28. Aitken J, Williams FL. A systematic review of thyroid dysfunction in preterm neonates exposed to topical iodine. Arch Dis Child Fetal Neonatal Ed 2014;99(1): F21–8.
29. Ahmet A, Lawson ML, Babyn P, et al. Hypothyroidism in neonates post-iodinated contrast media: a systematic review. Acta Paediatr 2009;98(10):1568–74.
30. Ares S, Quero J, de Escobar GM. Iodine balance, iatrogenic excess, and thyroid dysfunction in premature newborns. Semin Perinatol 2008;32(6):407–12.
31. Chan SS, Hams G, Wiley V, et al. Postpartum maternal iodine status and the relationship to neonatal thyroid function. Thyroid 2003;13(9):873–6.
32. Stathatos N, Levetan C, Burman KD, et al. The controversy of the treatment of critically ill patients with thyroid hormone. Best Pract Res Clin Endocrinol Metab 2001;15(4):465–78.
33. Peeters RP, Wouters PJ, van Toor H, et al. Serum 3,3',5'-triiodothyronine (rT3) and 3,5,3'-triiodothyronine/rT3 are prognostic markers in critically ill patients and are associated with postmortem tissue deiodinase activities. J Clin Endocrinol Metab 2005;90(8):4559–65.
34. Silva MH, Araujo MC, Diniz EM, et al. Nonthyroidal illnesses syndrome in full-term newborns with sepsis. Arch Endocrinol Metab 2015;59(6):528–34.
35. Stockigt JR. Guidelines for diagnosis and monitoring of thyroid disease: nonthyroidal illness. Clin Chem 1996;42(1):188–92.
36. Dilli D, Dilmen U. The role of interleukin-6 and C-reactive protein in non-thyroidal illness in premature infants followed in neonatal intensive care unit. J Clin Res Pediatr Endocrinol 2012;4(2):66–71.
37. Arai H, Goto R, Matsuda T, et al. Relationship between free T4 levels and postnatal steroid therapy in preterm infants. Pediatr Int 2009;51(6):800–3.
38. Filippi L, Pezzati M, Cecchi A, et al. Dopamine infusion: a possible cause of undiagnosed congenital hypothyroidism in preterm infants. Pediatr Crit Care Med 2006;7(3):249–51.
39. Lee JH, Kim SW, Jeon GW, et al. Thyroid dysfunction in very low birth weight preterm infants. Korean J Pediatr 2015;58(6):224–9.
40. Koulouri O, Moran C, Halsall D, et al. Pitfalls in the measurement and interpretation of thyroid function tests. Best Pract Res Clin Endocrinol Metab 2013;27(6): 745–62.
41. Gurnell M, Halsall DJ, Chatterjee VK. What should be done when thyroid function tests do not make sense? Clin Endocrinol 2011;74(6):673–8.
42. Stockigt JR, Lim CF. Medications that distort in vitro tests of thyroid function, with particular reference to estimates of serum free thyroxine. Best Pract Res Clin Endocrinol Metab 2009;23(6):753–67.
43. Alexander EK, Pearce EN, Brent GA, et al. 2017 guidelines of the American Thyroid Association for the diagnosis and management of thyroid disease during pregnancy and the postpartum. Thyroid 2017;27(3):315–89.
44. Mitchell ML, Hsu HW, Sahai I, et al. The increased incidence of congenital hypothyroidism: fact or fancy? Clin Endocrinol 2011;75(6):806–10.

45. Connelly KJ, Boston BA, Pearce EN, et al. Congenital hypothyroidism caused by excess prenatal maternal iodine ingestion. J Pediatr 2012;161(4):760–2.
46. Mengreli C, Kanaka-Gantenbein C, Girginoudis P, et al. Screening for congenital hypothyroidism: the significance of threshold limit in false-negative results. J Clin Endocrinol Metab 2010;95(9):4283–90.
47. Korada M, Pearce MS, Ward Platt MP, et al. Repeat testing for congenital hypothyroidism in preterm infants is unnecessary with an appropriate thyroid stimulating hormone threshold. Arch Dis Child Fetal Neonatal Ed 2008;93(4):F286–8.
48. van Wassenaer AG, Kok JH, de Vijlder JJ, et al. Effects of thyroxine supplementation on neurologic development in infants born at less than 30 weeks' gestation. N Engl J Med 1997;336(1):21–6.
49. Ng SM, Turner MA, Gamble C, et al. An explanatory randomised placebo controlled trial of levothyroxine supplementation for babies born <28 weeks' gestation: results of the TIPIT trial. Trials 2013;14:211.
50. van Wassenaer-Leemhuis A, Ares S, Golombek S, et al. Thyroid hormone supplementation in preterm infants born before 28 weeks gestational age and neurodevelopmental outcome at age 36 months. Thyroid 2014;24(7):1162–9.
51. Kawai M, Kusuda S, Cho K, et al. Nationwide surveillance of circulatory collapse associated with levothyroxine administration in very-low-birthweight infants in Japan. Pediatr Int 2012;54(2):177–81.
52. Delahunty C, Falconer S, Hume R, et al. Levels of neonatal thyroid hormone in preterm infants and neurodevelopmental outcome at 5 1/2 years: millennium cohort study. J Clin Endocrinol Metab 2010;95(11):4898–908.
53. Reuss ML, Paneth N, Pinto-Martin JA, et al. The relation of transient hypothyroxinemia in preterm infants to neurologic development at two years of age. N Engl J Med 1996;334(13):821–7.
54. Williams FL, Hume R. Perinatal factors affecting thyroid hormone status in extreme preterm infants. Semin Perinatol 2008;32(6):398–402.
55. Uchiyama A, Kushima R, Watanabe T, et al. Effect of l-thyroxine supplementation on infants with transient hypothyroxinemia of prematurity at 18 months of corrected age: randomized clinical trial. J Pediatr Endocrinol Metab 2015;28(1–2):177–82.
56. Uchiyama A, Kushima R, Watanabe T, et al. Effect of L-thyroxine supplementation on very low birth weight infants with transient hypothyroxinemia of prematurity at 3 years of age. J Perinatol 2017;37(5):602–5.

Neonatal Thyrotoxicosis

Stephanie L. Samuels, MD[a], Sisi M. Namoc, MD[b],
Andrew J. Bauer, MD[c],*

KEYWORDS

- Neonatal • Fetal • Thyrotoxicosis • Hyperthyroidism • Graves disease

KEY POINTS

- Neonatal thyrotoxicosis is most commonly caused by autoimmune hyperthyroidism, which results from transplacental passage of thyroid-stimulating hormone receptor–stimulating immunoglobulins from mother to fetus in the setting of maternal Graves disease.
- Pregnant women with current or past history of hyperthyroidism require screening to determine whether the fetus/neonate is at increased risk to develop hyperthyroidism.
- Nonautoimmune genetic causes of hyperthyroidism should be suspected in cases of neonatal thyrotoxicosis when there is no maternal history of Graves disease.
- Neonates with symptomatic hyperthyroidism require prompt initiation of therapy and close monitoring of response in consultation with a pediatric endocrinologist.

INTRODUCTION

Neonatal thyrotoxicosis (hyperthyroidism) is less prevalent than congenital hypothyroidism; however, it can lead to significant morbidity and mortality if not promptly recognized and adequately treated. Most cases are transient, secondary to maternal autoimmune hyperthyroidism (Graves disease [GD]). Neonatal hyperthyroidism can also occur secondary to activating mutations in the thyroid-stimulating hormone receptor (TSHR) or activating mutations in the stimulatory alpha subunit of the guanine nucleotide-binding protein (*GNAS*) gene in McCune-Albright (**Table 1**).

Disclosure: The authors do not have any commercial or financial conflicts of interested to report.

Funding: Research reported in this article for (S.L. Samuels) was supported by the National Center for Advancing Translational Sciences of the National Institutes of Health under award number TL1TR001880. The content is solely the responsibility of the authors and does not necessarily represent the official views of the National Institutes of Health.

[a] Division of Endocrinology and Diabetes, The Children's Hospital of Philadelphia, 3401 Civic Center Boulevard, Philadelphia, PA 19104, USA; [b] National Institute of Child Health, 600 Brasil Avenue, Breña - Lima 05, Peru; [c] Division of Endocrinology and Diabetes, The Children's Hospital of Philadelphia, The Thyroid Center, 3401 Civic Center Boulevard, Philadelphia, PA 19104, USA
* Corresponding author.
E-mail address: bauera@chop.edu

Clin Perinatol 45 (2018) 31–40
https://doi.org/10.1016/j.clp.2017.10.001
perinatology.theclinics.com

Table 1 Causes of neonatal hyperthyroidism		
Cause	**Cause**	**Expected Course**
Autoimmune hyperthyroidism (neonatal GD)	Transplacental passage of TRAb from mother to fetus	Transient (generally resolves in 4–5 mo after TRAb clearance)
Nonautoimmune hyperthyroidism	• Activating mutation in the TSH receptor (autosomal dominant) • Activating mutation in GNAS (McCune-Albright syndrome)	Permanent (persists after the neonatal period)

Abbreviation: TRAb, TSH receptor–stimulating antibodies.

This article summarizes current recommendations for screening and management of hyperthyroidism in both the fetal and neonatal periods, with a focus on neonatal thyrotoxicosis secondary to maternal GD. Early monitoring and treatment are crucial for optimizing short-term and long-term patient outcomes.

PATHOGENESIS OF NEONATAL HYPERTHYROIDISM
Neonatal Graves Disease

Neonatal GD is caused by transplacental passage of maternal stimulating TSHR antibodies (TRAb), leading to unregulated activation of the TSHR and overproduction of thyroid hormone. The prevalence of GD in pregnant women has been estimated to be about 0.1% to 0.4%, and studies have shown that approximately 1% to 5% of neonates born to mothers with GD develop hyperthyroidism.[1–3] Therefore, neonatal GD is expected to occur in 1 in 25,000 to 1 in 50,000 newborns. However, the incidence of neonatal GD may be higher if cases of asymptomatic biochemical hyperthyroidism are included.[4] Unlike GD in older children and adolescents, which disproportionately affects girls compared with boys, neonatal GD occurs in male and female infants equally.

Neonates of mothers with GD are at increased risk for neonatal GD, but hypothyroidism can also occur (**Fig. 1**). There are 2 types of TRAb: TSHR-stimulating immunoglobulins (TSI), which cause overproduction of thyroid hormone (hyperthyroidism), and TSHR inhibitory (blocking) immunoglobulins, which can cause hypothyroidism. Fetal thyroid hormone synthesis begins at approximately 10 to 12 weeks' gestation, and the fetal TSHR starts responding to stimulation, including stimulation by TSI, during the second trimester.[1] TRAb, which belong to the immunoglobulin G (IgG) class, freely cross the placenta, as does iodine, some thyroxine (T4), and any antithyroid drugs (ATDs) the mother may be taking for the treatment of GD. The balance of stimulatory and inhibitory TRAb, as well as ATD dose, influences the thyroid status in the fetus and neonate and the fluctuation of maternal antithyroid antibody titers may result in different risks to the fetus or neonate. One illustrative case report described a woman with GD whose 3 successive offspring had different outcomes: the first was euthyroid, the second developed transient hyperthyroidism, and the third was hypothyroid at birth.[5] In cases of neonatal GD, maternal TRAb typically clear from the infant's circulation by 4 to 6 months of age, with resultant resolution of hyperthyroidism.[1]

Other Causes

Nonautoimmune causes of neonatal hyperthyroidism, which are generally permanent rather than transient, have also been described. Genetic mutations causing constitutive activation of the *TSHR* are either inherited in an autosomal dominant manner or

Maternal Graves disease: Neonatal Thyroid Disorders

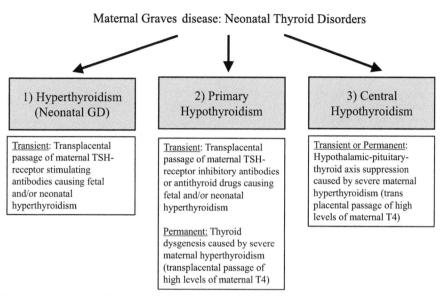

Fig. 1. Neonatal thyroid disorders in neonates of mothers with GD. T4, thyroxine.

may occur de novo, and lead to hyperthyroidism that may present during or after the neonatal period.[6,7] In McCune-Albright syndrome, activating mutations in *GNAS*, the gene encoding the alpha subunit of stimulatory G proteins, can also cause neonatal hyperthyroidism.[8] These genetic causes of neonatal hyperthyroidism should be considered in cases of neonatal thyrotoxicosis when there is no apparent maternal history of autoimmune hyperthyroidism.

Although iodine overload during pregnancy and during the neonatal period has frequently been associated with hypothyroidism, there is a theoretic potential for hyperthyroidism. Rare cases of thyrotoxicosis in a neonate following exposure to topical iodine have been reported.[9]

NEONATAL HYPERTHYROIDISM: FETAL ASPECTS
Manifestations of Hyperthyroidism in the Fetus

Signs of hyperthyroidism can be detected in the fetus, and, if present, are highly predictive of neonatal hyperthyroidism (**Box 1**). Particularly in cases in which maternal GD is poorly controlled, features concerning for fetal hyperthyroidism include fetal tachycardia (heart rate >160 beats/min), thyroid enlargement (goiter; fetal neck circumference >95%), intrauterine growth retardation, polyhydramnios or oligohydramnios, advanced bone age, craniosynostosis with microcephaly, and hydrops.[2,10] Polyhydramnios is typically associated with a goiter with resultant esophageal and/or tracheal obstruction. Fetal bone age is assessed at the distal femur, because the distal femoral epiphysis becomes detectable at about 32 weeks' gestation.[11] An advanced bone age is present if the femoral epiphysis is present before the 31st gestational week. For patients with severe thyrotoxicosis, there is an increased risk for premature delivery, and, at the extreme, fetal death may occur.[1]

Screening During Pregnancy

Recent consensus guidelines from the American Thyroid Association and Endocrine Society recommend determining maternal TRAb levels between 20 and 24 weeks'

Box 1
Manifestations of fetal and neonatal hyperthyroidism

Clinical manifestations of fetal hyperthyroidism:
- Tachycardia
- Goiter
- Intrauterine growth retardation
- Oligohydramnios
- Advanced bone maturation
- Prematurity
- Fetal death

Clinical manifestations of neonatal hyperthyroidism:
- Hemodynamic instability (tachycardia, hypertension, tachypnea/respiratory distress, hyperthermia)
- Irritability, sleep difficulty, hyperexcitability
- Increased appetite, feeding difficulties
- Poor weight gain or weight loss
- Diarrhea
- Flushing/sweating
- Stare and/or eyelid retardation
- Small fontanelle
- Craniosynostosis, microcephaly
- Severe cases: hepatosplenomegaly, thrombocytopenia, jaundice, pulmonary hypertension, cardiac failure, death

---

gestation.[12,13] All pregnant women with a history of GD, even those with hypothyroidism following definitive therapy with radioiodine ablation (RAI; ^{131}I) or total thyroidectomy, should undergo screening because increased TRAb levels can persist for years after definitive therapy. In a randomized controlled trial with 5-year follow-up, patients with newly diagnosed GD were randomized to receive medical therapy, thyroid surgery, or ^{131}I therapy. Medical therapy and surgery led to a disappearance of TRAb in 70% to 80% of patients after 18 months. In contrast, radioiodine (RAI) therapy led to increased TRAb levels over the first year following treatment and disappearance of TRAb was much less frequent, even years after RAI treatment.[14] Thus, all pregnant women taking thyroid hormone therapy for hypothyroidism should be asked whether they have a prior history of GD in order to determine which women should have TRAb testing in addition to the usual thyroid surveillance necessary to optimize levothyroxine therapy.

Pregnancies complicated by increased maternal TRAb levels are associated with a higher risk for development of fetal and neonatal hyperthyroidism. The risk increases markedly if maternal TRAb level is increased more than 2 to 3 times the upper limit of the normal range.[13] In one study of 35 infants born to mothers with GD, an increased maternal TRAb level 5 times greater than the normal range predicted neonatal thyrotoxicosis with a sensitivity of 100% and specificity of 76%.[15] In cases of poorly controlled maternal GD, maternal thyrotoxicosis can also cause central hypothyroidism, presumably through suppression of development of the fetal hypothalamic-pituitary-thyroid axis (see **Fig. 1**).[16] If maternal TRAb is negative during screening between 20 and 24 gestational weeks, and the mother is not on any ATD, then the baby is not at risk for development of neonatal GD and does not require any specific screening.

Early diagnosis of fetal hyperthyroidism can help prevent complications. Serial fetal ultrasonography, especially in cases of fetuses determined to be at increased risk based on high maternal TRAb level, should be performed by an experienced fetal ultrasonographer.[17,18] Nomograms for fetal thyroid gland surveillance have been developed.[19] Fetal ultrasonography should be completed at 20 weeks' gestation and then repeated every 4 to 6 weeks, particularly in cases of poorly controlled maternal hyperthyroidism.[10] It is important to distinguish fetal goiters caused by fetal hyperthyroidism from those caused by fetal hypothyroidism that may result from transplacental passage of maternal ATD. Examination of the vascularity of the goiter, as well as assessments of bone maturation and fetal heart rate, may guide determination of whether fetal hyperthyroidism or hypothyroidism is present.[10] Increased blood flow on Doppler ultrasonography imaging at the periphery of the thyroid is associated with hypothyroidism-induced goiter, and increased blood flow throughout the fetal goiter is associated with hyperthyroidism-induced fetal goiter.[17]

Management During Pregnancy

Pregnant women with hyperthyroidism/GD should be treated with medical therapy. Fetal hyperthyroidism can generally be prevented by adequate administration of ATDs to the mother. ATDs used for treatment of maternal GD include propylthiouracil (PTU) and methimazole (MMI), the active metabolite of carbimazole. The goal of therapy is to keep maternal free T4 (fT4) levels in the upper half of the normal range to maintain euthyroidism in the fetus.[13] Pregnant women with active GD should be treated with PTU rather than MMI during the first trimester, because of the increased risk for congenital anomalies associated with MMI.[12,13] A recent meta-analysis of 12 studies involving exposure to different ATDs during pregnancy found that exposure to MMI compared with PTU significantly increased the risk of neonatal congenital malformations.[20] Risks associated with MMI use include choanal or esophageal atresia, omphalomesenteric duct abnormalities, aplasia cutis, and dysmorphic facies. During the second and third trimesters, after the period linked with increased risk for congenital anomalies has passed, it is recommended that the ATD be switched from PTU to MMI because of increased risk for PTU-associated hepatotoxicity in the mother.[12]

RAI should not be administered to women attempting to conceive within 6 months of RAI treatment because of the increased risk of inducing neonatal or fetal hyperthyroidism secondary to RAI-increased maternal titers of TRAb or the risk of causing fetal hypothyroidism secondary to transplacental transport of the RAI. Surgical treatment would be favored as the definitive treatment before pregnancy but should only be considered during pregnancy if the mother has had a severe adverse reaction to ATD therapy or if very high doses of ATD are necessary (>30 mg/d of MMI or >450 mg/d of PTU), either secondary to refractory disease or to poor compliance. If surgery is required, the optimal timing is during the second trimester.[12,13]

Fetal hyperthyroidism can be managed by treatment of the mother with ATDs. In cases of maternal GD with TRAb positivity and suspected fetal hyperthyroidism, the maternal ATD dose may need to be increased to reduce fetal signs of hyperthyroidism. Normalization of fetal heart rate is a goal of maternal therapy. In contrast, if fetal hypothyroidism is suspected, the maternal ATD dose may need to be decreased.[10]

NEONATAL HYPERTHYROIDISM: NEONATAL ASPECTS
Manifestations of Hyperthyroidism in Neonates

Following birth, newborns may present with tachycardia, irritability with tremors, poor feeding, sweating, and difficulty sleeping secondary to thyrotoxicosis (see **Box 1**). Newborns may also have an emaciated appearance, proptosis with stare, and a goiter. Premature closure of cranial sutures (craniosynostosis) and subsequent microcephaly may be noted in severely affected infants. Other rare signs of neonatal hyperthyroidism that may be confused with infection/sepsis include thrombocytopenia, hepatosplenomegaly, and jaundice.[21] There have been reports of fulminant liver failure and pulmonary hypertension secondary to neonatal hyperthyroidism caused by maternal GD.[22–25]

In addition to having significant morbidity, neonates with hyperthyroidism are at increased risk for mortality without prompt treatment. In older case series, mortalities up to 12% to 20% have been reported, with cardiac failure the most common cause of death.[4]

Screening for Neonatal Hyperthyroidism

A screening algorithm for newborns at risk for neonatal thyrotoxicosis has been adapted from a recent review and is shown in **Fig. 2**.[26] Neonates considered to be at high risk for development of thyrotoxicosis include (1) infants born to mothers with GD, especially if the maternal TRAb level is great than 2 to 3 times the upper limit of normal; (2) infants in whom intrauterine surveillance revealed fetal signs of hyperthyroidism; and (3) infants with a known family history of genetic causes of congenital hyperthyroidism, including activating mutations in the TSHR (**Box 2**).

The algorithm in **Fig. 2** outlines recommended laboratory and clinical assessment for the first 2 weeks of life. If possible, TRAb levels should be determined in cord blood of infants at high risk for neonatal hyperthyroidism. Studies have shown strong correlations between maternal and neonatal TRAb levels. In one cohort study, 73% of newborns born to mothers with positive TRAb had increased cord blood TRAb levels, and 29% of these newborns subsequently developed neonatal hyperthyroidism.[27] Increased fT4 level between 3 and 7 days of life, but not at birth, was predictive of the development of hyperthyroidism in this study. Other studies have also shown that cord blood thyroid-stimulating hormone (TSH) and fT4 are less valuable in predicting onset of neonatal hyperthyroidism. Overall, the utility of cord blood TSH and fT4 levels in predicting onset of neonatal hyperthyroidism has not been established, and it is not recommended to obtain TSH and free T4 levels with cord blood.[26]

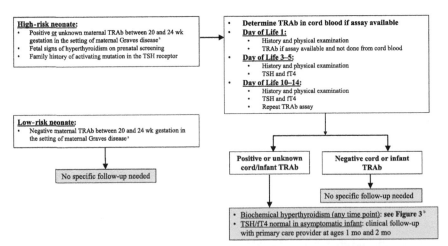

Fig. 2. Screening algorithm for newborns at risk for neonatal thyrotoxicosis. [a]Maternal TRAb level should be obtained in pregnant women with active or past GD/hyperthyroidism. [b]Neonates born to mothers with GD are also at risk for primary or central hypothyroidism and, in those cases, may require thyroid hormone replacement with levothyroxine. (*Adapted from* van der Kaay DC, Wasserman JD, Palmert MR. Management of neonates born to mothers with Graves' disease. Pediatrics 2016;137:e20151878.)

Box 2
Neonates at increased risk for thyrotoxicosis

Mother

- Increased TRAb/TSI levels during pregnancy
  ○ Active GD (hyperthyroidism)
  ○ Following treatment of GD with RAI
  ○ Following surgical treatment of GD (thyroidectomy)
- TRAb/TSI levels not assessed during pregnancy (unknown)
- ATD use during second/third trimester
- Clinical thyrotoxicosis during the second/third trimester
- Prior child with neonatal GD
- Family history of TSHR mutation

Baby

- Evidence of fetal thyrotoxicosis

Adapted from Ogilvy-Stuart AL. Neonatal thyroid disorders. Arch Dis Child Fetal Neonatal Ed 2002;87(3):F165–71.

If the neonate's TRAb level has not been obtained from cord blood, it should be determined as soon as possible after birth. Depending on how quickly TRAb results return from a particular laboratory, this level may not be available to inform clinical decision making. The newborn should be monitored closely for clinical and biochemical signs of overt hyperthyroidism. Maternal ATDs are usually metabolized and excreted by 5 days of life. Unless symptoms of hyperthyroidism develop earlier, thyroid function studies (TSH and fT4) should be sent between 3 and 5 days of life, when biochemical hyperthyroidism typically develops in neonates with hyperthyroidism secondary to maternal GD. Onset of signs and symptoms of thyrotoxicosis may be delayed for several days, either from the effect of maternal ATDs or because of the coexistent effect of blocking antibodies. Thyroid function studies should therefore be sent again at 10 to 14 days of life, because studies have shown that most cases of neonatal GD present within the first 2 weeks of life.[26] However, there have been case reports of overt thyrotoxicosis secondary to neonatal GD occurring as late as 45 days of life.[4] After 2 weeks of age, infants with no clinical or biochemical hyperthyroidism should continue close monthly follow-up with their primary care providers. Anticipatory guidance regarding signs of hyperthyroidism should be provided for parents.

Management of Neonatal Hyperthyroidism

A treatment algorithm for neonatal thyrotoxicosis has been adapted from a recent review (2016) and is shown in **Fig. 3**.[26] In cases of suspected neonatal GD with biochemical hyperthyroidism, MMI should be started at a dose of 0.2 to 0.5 mg/kg/d. Propranolol should be added at a dose of 2 mg/kg/d for signs of sympathetic hyperactivity, including tachycardia and hypertension. PTU is not recommended in neonates and throughout childhood because of the increased risk for hepatotoxicity.[28] In severe cases with hemodynamic compromise, Lugol solution or potassium iodide may be given. Glucocorticoids may also be beneficial in the short term. Because neonatal hyperthyroidism is transient and resolves with clearance of maternal TRAb from the circulation, thyroid function tests should be monitored closely every 1 to 2 weeks following initiation of treatment to ensure appropriate MMI dose titration.[26]

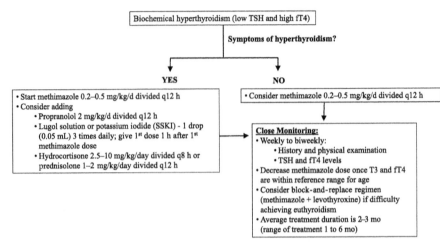

Fig. 3. Management for neonates with thyrotoxicosis. q, every; T3, triiodothyronine. (*Adapted from* van der Kaay DC, Wasserman JD, Palmert MR. Management of neonates born to mothers with Graves' disease. Pediatrics 2016;137:e20151878.)

The benefit of treatment of asymptomatic biochemical hyperthyroidism has not been shown as clearly.[26]

In cases of nonautoimmune neonatal hyperthyroidism (activating mutations of the TSHR or McCune-Albright syndrome), MMI should be used for treatment similarly to cases of neonatal GD. Definitive therapy, including thyroidectomy and/or RAI will ultimately be required but can be delayed for months to years if the baby is responsive to medical therapy.[29,30]

Current guidelines note that breastfeeding is safe for mothers on antithyroid medications, at moderate doses of MMI (20–30 mg/d) and PTU (<300 mg/d).[31] Infants of mothers with GD who are breastfeeding should have periodic thyroid function screening to ensure they have not developed hypothyroidism. In one study of 42 breastfeeding mothers with hyperthyroidism treated with moderate doses of MMI, no significant differences in growth or intellectual development were seen in children at follow-up at age 48 to 84 months.[32]

OUTCOMES OF NEONATAL THYROTOXICOSIS

In addition to the well-documented short-term consequences, there is some evidence to suggest that there are long-term negative outcomes of neonatal thyrotoxicosis, particularly if inadequately treated. Normal thyroid hormone levels are important for normal brain development, and the adverse neurocognitive effects of congenital hypothyroidism are well known. In contrast, studies of neurocognitive outcomes of infants with thyrotoxicosis are limited. One study of 8 children with histories of neonatal thyrotoxicosis showed intellectual impairment and craniosynostosis in 6 children and intellectual impairment in 4 children at age 2 years or older.[33] Another study of 17 children of hyperthyroid mothers receiving ATDs during pregnancy showed no effects of ATD treatment on thyroid gland size/function or physical and intellectual development after the neonatal period.[34] Further studies are needed to assess whether neonatal hyperthyroidism leads to long-term complications. Results will help inform management strategies in order to optimize patient outcomes.

SUMMARY

Infants at risk for development of neonatal hyperthyroidism benefit from a multidisciplinary approach to care beginning prenatally, including a team of obstetricians and radiologists with expertise in maternal-fetal medicine, neonatologists, pediatricians, and pediatric endocrinologists. Quality improvement initiatives should be designed to ensure proper implementation of screening guidelines for pregnant women with hyperthyroidism as well as appropriate screening and management for fetal/neonatal hyperthyroidism. Early diagnosis and commencement of therapy is necessary to prevent short-term and potential long-term adverse outcomes of neonatal thyrotoxicosis. Future studies are needed to assess the long-term effects of neonatal thyrotoxicosis, including impacts on thyroid function, growth, and cognitive development.

REFERENCES

1. Polak M, Legac I, Vuillard E, et al. Congenital hyperthyroidism: the fetus as a patient. Horm Res 2006;65(5):235–42.
2. Zimmerman D. Fetal and neonatal hyperthyroidism. Thyroid 1999;9(7):727–33.
3. Cooper DS, Laurberg P. Hyperthyroidism in pregnancy. Lancet Diabetes Endocrinol 2013;1(3):238–49.
4. Ogilvy-Stuart AL. Neonatal thyroid disorders. Arch Dis Child Fetal Neonatal Ed 2002;87(3):F165–71.
5. Fort P, Lifshitz F, Pugliese M, et al. Neonatal thyroid disease: differential expression in three successive offspring. J Clin Endocrinol Metab 1988;66(3):645–7.
6. Watkins MG, Dejkhamron P, Huo J, et al. Persistent neonatal thyrotoxicosis in a neonate secondary to a rare thyroid-stimulating hormone receptor activating mutation: case report and literature review. Endocr Pract 2008;14(4):479–83.
7. Chester J, Rotenstein D, Ringkananont U, et al. Congenital neonatal hyperthyroidism caused by germline mutations in the TSH receptor gene. J Pediatr Endocrinol Metab 2008;21(5):479–86.
8. Lourenco R, Dias P, Gouveia R, et al. Neonatal McCune-Albright syndrome with systemic involvement: a case report. J Med Case Rep 2015;9:189.
9. Bryant WP, Zimmerman D. Iodine-induced hyperthyroidism in a newborn. Pediatrics 1995;95(3):434–6.
10. Leger J. Management of fetal and neonatal Graves' disease. Horm Res Paediatr 2017;87(1):1–6.
11. Goldstein I, Lockwood C, Belanger K, et al. Ultrasonographic assessment of gestational age with the distal femoral and proximal tibial ossification centers in the third trimester. Am J Obstet Gynecol 1988;158(1):127–30.
12. Alexander EK, Pearce EN, Brent GA, et al. 2017 guidelines of the American Thyroid Association for the diagnosis and management of thyroid disease during pregnancy and the postpartum. Thyroid 2017;27(3):315–89.
13. De Groot L, Abalovich M, Alexander EK, et al. Management of thyroid dysfunction during pregnancy and postpartum: an Endocrine Society clinical practice guideline. J Clin Endocrinol Metab 2012;97(8):2543–65.
14. Laurberg P, Wallin G, Tallstedt L, et al. TSH-receptor autoimmunity in Graves' disease after therapy with anti-thyroid drugs, surgery, or radioiodine: a 5-year prospective randomized study. Eur J Endocrinol 2008;158(1):69–75.
15. Peleg D, Cada S, Peleg A, et al. The relationship between maternal serum thyroid-stimulating immunoglobulin and fetal and neonatal thyrotoxicosis. Obstet Gynecol 2002;99(6):1040–3.

16. Kempers MJ, van Tijn DA, van Trotsenburg AS, et al. Central congenital hypothyroidism due to gestational hyperthyroidism: detection where prevention failed. J Clin Endocrinol Metab 2003;88(12):5851–7.
17. Luton D, Le Gac I, Vuillard E, et al. Management of Graves' disease during pregnancy: the key role of fetal thyroid gland monitoring. J Clin Endocrinol Metab 2005;90(11):6093–8.
18. Polak M, Le Gac I, Vuillard E, et al. Fetal and neonatal thyroid function in relation to maternal Graves' disease. Best Pract Res Clin Endocrinol Metab 2004;18(2): 289–302.
19. Ranzini AC, Ananth CV, Smulian JC, et al. Ultrasonography of the fetal thyroid: nomograms based on biparietal diameter and gestational age. J Ultrasound Med 2001;20(6):613–7.
20. Song R, Lin H, Chen Y, et al. Effects of methimazole and propylthiouracil exposure during pregnancy on the risk of neonatal congenital malformations: a meta-analysis. PLoS One 2017;12(7):e0180108.
21. Neal PR, Jansen RD, Lemons JA, et al. Unusual manifestations of neonatal hyperthyroidism. Am J Perinatol 1985;2(3):231–5.
22. Loomba-Albrecht LA, Bremer AA, Wong A, et al. Neonatal cholestasis caused by hyperthyroidism. J Pediatr Gastroenterol Nutr 2012;54(3):433–4.
23. Hasosah M, Alsaleem K, Qurashi M, et al. Neonatal hyperthyroidism with fulminant liver failure: a case report. J Clin Diagn Res 2017;11(4):SD01–2.
24. Oden J, Cheifetz IM. Neonatal thyrotoxicosis and persistent pulmonary hypertension necessitating extracorporeal life support. Pediatrics 2005;115(1):e105–8.
25. Obeid R, Kalra VK, Arora P, et al. Neonatal thyrotoxicosis presenting as persistent pulmonary hypertension. BMJ Case Rep 2012;2012 [pii:bcr0220125939].
26. van der Kaay DC, Wasserman JD, Palmert MR. Management of neonates born to mothers with Graves' disease. Pediatrics 2016;137(4) [pii:e20151878].
27. Besancon A, Beltrand J, Le Gac I, et al. Management of neonates born to women with Graves' disease: a cohort study. Eur J Endocrinol 2014;170(6):855–62.
28. Rivkees SA, Stephenson K, Dinauer C. Adverse events associated with methimazole therapy of graves' disease in children. Int J Pediatr Endocrinol 2010;2010: 176970.
29. Paschke R, Niedziela M, Vaidya B, et al. 2012 European Thyroid Association guidelines for the management of familial and persistent sporadic nonautoimmune hyperthyroidism caused by thyroid-stimulating hormone receptor germline mutations. Eur Thyroid J 2012;1(3):142–7.
30. Mastorakos G, Mitsiades NS, Doufas AG, et al. Hyperthyroidism in McCune-Albright syndrome with a review of thyroid abnormalities sixty years after the first report. Thyroid 1997;7(3):433–9.
31. Speller E, Brodribb W. Breastfeeding and thyroid disease: a literature review. Breastfeed Rev 2012;20(2):41–7.
32. Azizi F. Treatment of post-partum thyrotoxicosis. J Endocrinol Invest 2006;29(3): 244–7.
33. Daneman D, Howard NJ. Neonatal thyrotoxicosis: intellectual impairment and craniosynostosis in later years. J Pediatr 1980;97(2):257–9.
34. Messer PM, Hauffa BP, Olbricht T, et al. Antithyroid drug treatment of Graves' disease in pregnancy: long-term effects on somatic growth, intellectual development and thyroid function of the offspring. Acta Endocrinol (Copenh) 1990;123(3): 311–6.

Neonatal Diabetes Mellitus
An Update on Diagnosis and Management

Michelle Blanco Lemelman, MD[a], Lisa Letourneau, MPH, RD, LDN[b],
Siri Atma W. Greeley, MD, PhD[c],*

KEYWORDS

- Neonatal diabetes • Monogenic diabetes • Genetic • Insulin • Glyburide

---

INTRODUCTION

Diabetes mellitus most commonly occurs after the neonatal period and results from complex interactions between both environmental and incompletely penetrant genetic factors. Advances in molecular genetics over the past decade hastened the realization that diabetes that occurs very early life is most often due to underlying monogenic defects, disorders caused by mutations in a single gene. Neonatal (or congenital) diabetes mellitus (NDM) is now known to occur in approximately 1 in 90,000 to 160,000 live births.[1] There are more than 20 known genetic causes for NDM.

NDM may be categorized by phenotypic characteristics into transient, permanent, and syndromic forms. In a large international cohort study of 1020 patients clinically diagnosed with diabetes before 6 months of age, 80% had a known genetic diagnosis.[2] Mutations in *KCNJ11* and *ABCC8* (affecting the pancreatic beta-cell potassium [K]-ATP channel) may be treated with oral sulfonylureas (SUs) and account for about 40% of these patients. Preliminary studies indicate that early SU treatment, in contrast to insulin, may improve neurodevelopmental outcomes in SU-responsive patients.[3] It is important to diagnose monogenic diabetes as early as possible, as it can predict the clinical course, explain additional clinical features, and guide appropriate management for patients.[4]

HYPERGLYCEMIA IN THE NEONATAL PERIOD

Although neonatal diabetes may be recognized within the first few days of life, there are alternative causes of hyperglycemia in neonates, which can make the diagnosis of diabetes difficult. This difficulty is especially true in the preterm or

---

Disclosures: The authors have no financial or commercial relationships to disclose.
[a] Section of Adult and Pediatric Endocrinology, Diabetes, and Metabolism, MC 5053, 5841 South Maryland Avenue, Chicago, IL 60637, USA; [b] Monogenic Diabetes Registry, University of Chicago Medicine, Kovler Diabetes Center, 900 East 57th Street, Chicago, IL 60637, USA; [c] Section of Adult and Pediatric Endocrinology, Diabetes, and Metabolism, Kovler Diabetes Center, The University of Chicago, 900 East 57th Street, Chicago, IL 60637, USA
* Corresponding author.
E-mail address: sgreeley@peds.bsd.uchicago.edu

low-birth-weight infant.[5] The prevalence of high glucose levels in preterm infants is 25% to 75%.[6,7] Neonatal hyperglycemia is more common in the first 3 to 5 days after birth but can be found in infants at up to 10 days of life; it usually resolves within 2 to 3 days of onset.[8]

Typical causes for hyperglycemia in this group include increased parenteral glucose administration, sepsis, increased counter-regulatory hormones due to stress, and medications, such as steroids.[8] There is some evidence of insufficient pancreatic insulin secretion and relative insulin resistance in hyperglycemic and nonhyperglycemic critically ill preterm neonates.[6,9] However, there is no clear consensus related to the treatment of neonatal hyperglycemia; many institutions may follow personalized approaches. In the neonatal intensive care unit at the University of Chicago, patients are commonly placed on insulin when point-of-care dextrose persistently reaches 300 mg/dL or greater. Related literature suggests that intervention may be warranted when blood sugar levels are greater than 180 mg/dL. However, because of the low risk of short-term hyperglycemia in neonates and the high risk of insulin-induced hypoglycemia, Rozance and Hay[8] recommend reserving insulin therapy for severe hyperglycemia, defined as glucose levels greater than 500 mg/dL. Another consideration is that significant osmotic changes leading to ventricular hemorrhage may occur at glucose levels greater than 360 mg/dL.[9] Regardless of the cause of hyperglycemia, the authors recommend intervention with insulin when glucose levels are persistently more than 250 mg/dL. Irrespective of the glucose threshold, patients with persistent elevations should be started on an intravenous insulin infusion, although in some circumstances subcutaneous insulin could be considered (discussed in detail later).

Term infants and premature infants born at greater than 32 weeks' gestational age (GA) are more likely to have a monogenic cause for their diabetes than are very premature infants born at less than 32 weeks' GA.[5] However, according to the same study, 31% of all preterm infants with diabetes born at less than 32 weeks' GA were diagnosed with a monogenic cause, strongly suggesting that such infants should have genetic testing.[5] These preterm infants also tend to present earlier with diabetes (around 1 week of age) compared with full-term infants (around 6 weeks of age). Data gathered from the Monogenic Diabetes Registry at the University of Chicago and others show that patients with transient forms of neonatal diabetes present earlier on average (most often within days of birth) as compared with those with permanent forms.[1,10,11]

NDM should be considered in infants with insulin-dependent hyperglycemia, with blood glucoses persistently greater than 250 mg/dL, without an alternative cause. Neonatologists should become suspicious of diabetes when hyperglycemia persists for longer than 7 to 10 days. Some literature alternatively suggests pursuing genetic testing when hyperglycemia persists beyond the first 2 to 3 weeks of life.[9] However, genetic testing should be sent immediately in patients who present with acute extreme hyperglycemia (serum glucose >1000 mg/dL) without an identified cause, regardless of the time course. Of note, some forms of NDM, such as 6q24, may be transient, presenting only for a few days to weeks before resolving. The authors recommend sending genetic testing immediately, even if hyperglycemia resolves.

The initial assessment of children with suspected disease should include laboratory assessment of urine ketones, serum glucose, C peptide, and insulin. A pancreatic ultrasound should be performed, as the presence or absence of a pancreas will guide diagnosis and therapy considerations. The timing of the appearance of diabetes-related autoantibodies in neonates has not been well studied. Literature analyzing antibodies in the offspring of parents with type 1 diabetes (T1D) conclude that maternal antibodies may be present in the neonate for up to 6 months. In addition, specific detection of insulin antibodies after 6 months of age was associated with developing disease.[12] The authors would, therefore, suggest that testing for autoantibodies within the first 6 months of life will not change the decision about mandatory genetic testing and, thus, may not be essential.

Neonatal diabetes may not always present in the immediate neonatal period. More recent studies show that monogenic forms of NDM may still occur at up to 12 months of age, albeit at a reduced frequency.[1,13] The likelihood of monogenic diabetes causing hyperglycemia in children older than 12 months of age is much lower. Patients may present insidiously (with polyuria, polydipsia, or failure to thrive), acutely (with ketoacidosis or altered mental status), or incidentally without symptoms.[14]

The odds of presenting with diabetic ketoacidosis (DKA) increases with age; this is likely the result of the difficulty recognizing early signs of diabetes in infancy.[1] Currently there is very little published regarding presenting signs and symptoms of diabetes in infancy. A recent study at the University of Chicago reported that 66.2% of subjects with monogenic diabetes, of all types, presented with DKA.[1] When patients present between 6 and 12 months of life, monogenic diabetes is less likely; but genetic testing should still be pursued. Antibodies for T1D should be drawn, including glutamate decarboxylase, zinc transporter-8, insulin, and islet antigen-2 autoantibodies. Laboratory assessment should also include urine and serum ketones, serum glucose, serum insulin, and C-peptide levels. Incidence studies in Europe show that the number of predicted new cases of T1D in the zero to 5-year age group will double by the year 2020.[15] Making the distinction of neonatal diabetes from T1D as early as possible is paramount for management and treatment decisions.

TYPES OF DIABETES

Prognosis and treatment options for monogenic forms of NDM depend heavily on which gene is affected. Advances in genetic testing have allowed for more efficient and comprehensive testing to be readily available.[16] Despite the fact that genetic testing is expensive, in the case of neonatal diabetes, it is clearly cost-effective largely because of the high proportion of patients whose treatment will improve by such testing.[17] Therefore, genetic testing is indicated for all cases of diabetes diagnosed at less than 12 months of age. Here the authors provide details on some of the most common forms of infancy-onset diabetes (**Table 1**).

KCNJ11, ABCC8

Activating heterozygous mutations in the genes encoding either of the subunits of the ATP-sensitive K channel (K_{ATP} channel; *KCNJ11* or *ABCC8*) of the pancreatic beta-cell are the most common causes of permanent neonatal diabetes and the second most common cause of transient NDM.[2] Combined, these mutations account for more than 50% of all cases of NDM.[18]

Mechanism of action
In the normal pancreatic beta-cell, increased glucose across the GLUT 2 transporter is metabolized by the enzyme glucokinase, resulting in increased production of ATP. This causes closure of the K_{ATP} channel, which, in turn, depolarizes the cell membrane, activating the influx of calcium through voltage-gated calcium channels that subsequently allows for exocytosis of insulin granules. *KCNJ11* encodes for the inner subunit (Kir6.2) of the K_{ATP} channel, whereas *ABCC8* encodes for the outer subunit (SUR1). Mutations in either gene cause the K_{ATP} channels to remain inappropriately stuck open even in the presence of hyperglycemia. Without channel closure, the cell membrane is not able to depolarize effectively; thus, insulin cannot be released from the beta-cell.

Table 1
All known monogenic causes of neonatal diabetes with associated features, from more common to less common (top to bottom)

Gene	Transient vs Permanent	Inheritance	Features	Treatment
KCNJ11	Either	Spontaneous (80%), AD (20%)	Low birthweight, developmental delay, seizures (DEND syndrome), may have other neurologic features	Insulin SU
ABCC8	Either	Spontaneous, AD	Low birthweight	Insulin SU
6q24	Transient	Spontaneous, AD for paternal duplications	Low birth weight, possible IUGR, diagnosed earlier than channel mutations (closer to birth), relapsed cases may respond to SU	Insulin
INS	Either	Spontaneous (80%), AD (20%) AR (rare: T or P)	Low birthweight	Insulin
GATA6	Permanent	Spontaneous, AD	Pancreatic hypoplasia or agenesis, exocrine insufficiency, cardiac defect	Insulin
EIF2AK3[a]	Permanent	Spontaneous, AR	Wolcott-Rallison syndrome, skeletal dysplasia (1–2 y old) Episodic acute liver failure, exocrine pancreatic insufficiency	Insulin
GCK[a]	Permanent	Spontaneous, AR (neonatal diabetes), AD (GCK-MODY)	Low birthweight	Insulin
PTF1A	Permanent	Spontaneous, AR	Neurologic abnormalities, exocrine insufficiency, kidney involvement	Insulin
FOXP3	Permanent	X-linked	Autoimmune thyroid disease, exfoliative dermatitis, enteropathy (IPEX syndrome)	Insulin
ZFP57	Transient	Spontaneous, maternal Hypomethylation Imprinting	Variable phenotype Low birth weight, macroglossia, developmental delay	Insulin
GLIS3[a]	Permanent	Spontaneous, AR	Hypothyroidism, kidney cysts, glaucoma, hepatic fibrosis	Insulin

(continued on next page)

	Table 1 (*continued*)			
Gene	**Transient vs Permanent**	**Inheritance**	**Features**	**Treatment**
PDX1	Permanent	Spontaneous, AR (neonatal diabetes), AD (PDX1-MODY)	Pancreatic hypoplasia or agenesis, exocrine insufficiency	Insulin
SLC2A2	Either	Spontaneous, AR	Fanconi-Bickel syndrome (hepatomegaly, RTA)	Insulin
SLC19A2	Permanent	Spontaneous, AR	Neurologic deficit (stroke, seizure) Visual disturbance; cardiac abnormality	Insulin Thiamine (rarely)
GATA4	Permanent	Spontaneous, AR	Pancreatic hypoplasia or agenesis, exocrine insufficiency, cardiac defect	Insulin
NEUROD1	Permanent	Spontaneous, AR	Neurologic abnormalities (later), learning difficulties, sensorineural deafness	Insulin
NEUROG3	Permanent	Spontaneous, AR	Diarrhea (due to lack of enteroendocrine cells)	Insulin
NKX2-2	Permanent		Neurologic abnormalities (later), very low birth weight	Insulin
RFX6[a]	Permanent	Spontaneous, AR	Low birthweight, intestinal atresia, gall bladder hypoplasia, diarrhea	Insulin
IER3IP1[a]	Permanent	Spontaneous, AR	Microcephaly, infantile epileptic encephalopathy	Insulin
MNX1[a]	Permanent	Spontaneous, AR	Neurologic abnormalities (later)	Insulin
HNF1B	Transient	Spontaneous, AD	Pancreatic atrophy, abnormal kidney, and genitalia development	Insulin

Abbreviations: AD, autosomal dominant; AR, autosomal recessive; DEND, developmental delay, epilepsy, and neonatal diabetes; DM, diabetes mellitus; IUGR, intrauterine growth restriction; MODY, maturity onset diabetes of the young; RTA, renal tubular acidosis; SGA, small for gestational age.

[a] Autosomal recessive forms may be more likely in populations or families with known consanguinity.

Presentation

Although *KCNJ11/ABCC8* mutations typically lead to the onset of diabetes before 6 months of age, a diagnosis after 6 months is also possible. In a recent study of subjects diagnosed at less than 1 year of age, the median age at diagnosis for subjects with *KCNJ11/ABCC8* was 9.6 weeks (interquartile range [IQR] 6.1–18.3 weeks).[1]

Estimates of DKA frequency at the diagnosis vary between 30% and 75%.[1,19,20] Intrauterine growth restriction (thus, small-for-gestational age birthweight) is common in patients with these conditions.

Treatment

Although many patients may be managed with insulin during the initial hospitalization and diagnosis, most patients with mutations in these genes can be treated with high-dose SU medications (typically 0.5–1.0 mg/kg/d of glyburide or even greater, depending mostly on the specific mutation). SUs act on the K_{ATP} channel to promote closure, allowing for insulin to be released from the beta-cell. The use of SUs in pediatric patients is considered an off-label use and is discussed later in more detail.

Associated features

Because of the presence of K_{ATP} channels in the brain, patients with mutations in *KCNJ11*, particularly those with permanent forms, may exhibit increased frequency of attention-deficit/ hyperactivity disorder, sleep disruptions, developmental delays, and seizures.[21,22] Effects may vary from mild delays without seizures to more severe delays with seizures (developmental delay, epilepsy, and neonatal diabetes [DEND] syndrome). Patients with certain mutations may have such mild delays that they remain unnoticed by their caregivers and health care providers until they emerge later in life as specific deficits become apparent when compared with their unaffected siblings.[21] SU therapy may improve neurologic function in addition to improving glycemic control,[23–25] and earlier initiation of SUs may offer more benefit.[3] These associations have not been as well characterized in patients with permanent *ABCC8* mutations or in transient forms of either gene.

6q24-Related Neonatal Diabetes Mellitus

Overexpression of genes at chromosome 6q24 is the most common cause of transient neonatal diabetes.[26]

Mechanism of action

This NDM disorder can occur through any of 3 distinct mechanisms (**Fig. 1**), most often epigenetic: uniparental disomy of chromosome 6 (in which there are only 2 copies of 6q24 but both come from the father), duplication of the paternal 6q24 allele (in which there are 3 copies of 6q24, but 2 are from the father), or loss of maternal methylation (in which there is a defect in the silencing of the maternal allele, which can be recessively inherited). Paternal duplications are autosomal dominant and, thus, carry a 50% transmission risk when inherited from the father.[27]

Presentation

Patients with 6q24-related NDM typically present within the first few days or weeks of life,[28] usually without DKA.[1] Although the patients' hyperglycemia may go away within the first year or so of life, hypoglycemia is possible during the remission period.[29] Although the exact risk is uncertain, it seems to be highly likely that the hyperglycemia will return during the teenage years; this persists into adulthood in most cases.[28]

Treatment

Insulin is typically used during the early neonatal phase, although there is a possibility of a response to SU in some cases.[30] The best treatment option during the later relapse phase remains unclear; but these patients have been shown to have the ability to produce insulin and, thus, should not be treated as though they have T1D. Although

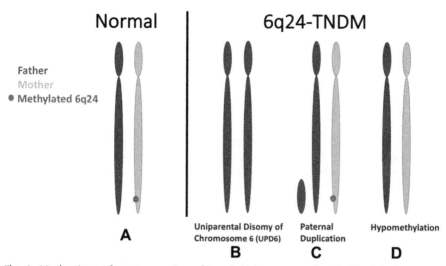

Normal | 6q24-TNDM

Father
Mother
● Methylated 6q24

A

Uniparental Disomy of
Chromosome 6 (UPD6)
B

Paternal
Duplication
C

Hypomethylation
D

Fig. 1. Mechanisms of overexpression of imprinted genes causing 6q24-related neonatal diabetes. Diabetes in all cases results from overexpression of genes that are normally either silenced by maternal methylation or expressed when paternally inherited (*A*). Overexpression, thus, occurs when (*B*) both copies are paternally inherited in uniparental paternal disomy (UPD6, which can be either complete disomy or hetero-disomy), (*C*) an additional copy is paternally inherited because of a duplication that includes 6q24, or (*D*) there is a defect in maternal methylation (which can be due to recessive mutations in ZFP57). Although the parent of origin determination or detection of duplication can be possible through a variety of methods, the most comprehensive direct way of testing of overexpression of genes at 6q24 from any cause is methylation-specific multiplex ligation-dependent probe amplification or methylation-specific polymerase chain reaction/sequencing-based and is rarely offered in most commercial laboratories.

insulin has often been used in these older patients, recent studies have shown that noninsulin therapies used for type 2 diabetes may be highly effective.[31,32]

Associated features
Patients with 6q24-related neonatal diabetes may also present with macroglossia or umbilical hernia.

Insulin Gene

Alterations in the insulin gene (*INS*) are the second most common cause of permanent neonatal diabetes.[33]

Mechanism of action
Mutations in the insulin gene seem in most cases to lead to misfolding of the insulin protein. These proteins accumulate in various subcellular compartments and seem to increase endoplasmic reticulum (ER) stress and subsequent beta-cell death.[34–36]

Presentation
Patients with *INS* mutations may appear clinically similar to patients with early onset T1D. Although most cases will be diagnosed before 6 months of age, cases diagnosed near 12 months of age and even into the toddler years have been reported. Letourneau and colleagues[1] found a median age at diagnosis of 10 weeks (IQR 6.1–17.4) with 30% presenting in DKA.

Treatment

Patients will require insulin therapy. Anecdotal evidence suggests that early, aggressive treatment with insulin may help to preserve some beta-cell function.

Associated features

No other specific features are known to be associated with *INS*-related neonatal diabetes.

Less Common Forms

Mutations in more than 20 genes are now known to cause diabetes onset within the first year of life, but most of these are exceedingly rare recessive conditions. Among these rarer causes, a few are relatively more common and are worth mentioning, because early recognition of associated features can be important for long-term outcomes.

GATA6, PDX1

GATA6 and PDX1 are transcription factors critical to pancreatic development. Mutations in either gene can result in a varying degree of pancreatic hypoplasia, including possible complete agenesis.[37] Insulin therapy, as well as pancreatic enzyme replacement therapy, is necessary for appropriate growth and glycemic control.

EIF2AK3

Homozygous mutations in *EIF2AK3* induce ER stress and, thus, beta-cell death and are the most common cause of NDM among consanguineous families.[2] Several other features may include episodic hepatic dysfunction and skeletal dysplasia; however, because these are not usually apparent in the neonatal phase, early genetic testing will help guide monitoring and management.[38] Insulin treatment is required.

FOXP3

Mutations in *FOXP3* cause a monogenic form of autoimmune diabetes, most often as part of the immune dysregulation, polyendocrinopathy, enteropathy, X-linked (IPEX) syndrome..[39,40] Because the associated features of IPEX are severe enough to often cause death within the first year of life, stem cell transplantation is often considered. Early genetic diagnosis would be essential in guiding clinical decision-making.

Early Onset Autoimmune Type 1 Diabetes

Most patients diagnosed with diabetes after 6 months of age will have autoimmune T1D. Among subjects diagnosed at less than 1 year of age, those with likely T1D had a median diagnosis at 42.6 weeks of age (IQR 37.4–50.4) and 87.5% presented in DKA at diagnosis.[1] They may be less likely to have a low birth weight. Most of these patients will test positive for at least one diabetes autoantibody. For those who have a negative autoantibody and/or genetic testing, a T1D genetic risk score assessment (most often done on a research basis) may be helpful to discern the true cause.[37] There is some evidence to suggest that patients with early onset T1D may experience more aggressive beta-cell decline than those diagnosed at older ages.

MANAGEMENT CONSIDERATIONS

The initial approach to hyperglycemia includes assessing the quantity of glucose being administered and reducing the glucose infusion rate when it does not affect patients' nutrition and growth. In the neonate, ideal glucose infusion rates should be 6 to 12 mg/kg/min to maintain appropriate minimums for growth without inefficient conversion of energy to fat.[9] Patients with hyperglycemia are initially managed on an intravenous insulin infusion. Guidelines for dosing and titrating insulin infusions in neonates are lacking in the literature. In studies assessing early insulin therapy in very-low-birth-weight infants, an initial dosage of 0.05 units per kilogram per hour was commonly used.[6] However, other studies show effective glucose control with insulin rates ranging as low as 0.02 units per kilogram per hour, much lower than the standard dosage of 0.1 units per kilogram per hour used in older children in DKA.[41] In infancy, insulin infusion rates should be titrated by small increments of 0.01 units per kilogram per hour in response to glucose levels less than 200 (decrease infusion rate) or greater than 250 mg/dL (increase infusion rate). However, dosing should ultimately be guided by clinical judgment. The capillary blood glucose (BG) level should be monitored at least every hour while on intravenous insulin infusion. When hyperglycemia is persistent and insulin dependence is established, the provider should consider transition to subcutaneous insulin injections, in part to avoid complications related to central venous catheters. Treatment should be guided by recommendations from a pediatric endocrinologist.

Subcutaneous Insulin

The initial subcutaneous doses of insulin should be given conservatively, when BG levels are at least greater than 200 to 250 mg/dL. The authors would recommend starting with preprandial short-acting doses in the amount of 0.1 to 0.15 units per kilogram per dose or doses guided by the response to intravenous insulin. The dose should be given before feeds when blood sugars are greater than 200 to 250 mg/dL. Because of the frequency of oral intake in newborns, insulin should only be given preprandially. All preprandial blood sugars should be checked at least initially, but insulin doses may only be needed with every other feed (3–4 times per day). The smallest, feasible subcutaneous dose of any insulin, including long acting (glargine) and short acting (lispro or aspart), without dilution is 0.5 units.

Smaller doses of U-100 (100 units of insulin per 1 milliliter of liquid) that would otherwise be immeasurable are possible by dilution, preferably with an insulin-specific compatible diluent (typically available through the manufacturers). Diluting one part of aspart or lispro to 9 parts diluent will yield a concentration of one-tenth of the original concentration (U-10). Therefore, doses of 0.1 to 0.9 U-100 may be used as subcutaneous injections. Such a preparation of lispro may be used for up to 28 days when stored at 41°F (and up to 14 days when stored at 86°F),[42] whereas the preparation of aspart may be used for up to 28 days when stored at 86°F or less.[43] Of note, U-10 insulin aspart may be stable for up to 7 days at 98.6°F or less when used in a continuous subcutaneous insulin infusion (CSII) pump (insulin pump).[44] However, diluted insulin is typically not necessary for use with insulin pumps because they are capable of administering very small doses of U-100 preparations (see later discussion). Clinical personnel, patients, and families should use caution with diluted preparations in the hospital and at home because of the potential for dosing errors.

Whether using diluted or undiluted insulin subcutaneously, the authors would recommend against the use of intermediate-acting insulins, such as regular and NPH, which have been associated with an increased risk of hypoglycemia compared with short- and long-acting analogues.[45] Although infants are feeding frequently and clinicians may be tempted to cover basal and bolus requirements with an intermediate insulin, when the feeding schedule ultimately becomes more spaced out, these infants will be at a higher risk of hypoglycemia. Just as with older patients, infants should also be placed on a regimen of multiple daily injections of insulin (MDI) with daily or twice-daily long-acting insulin and multiple daily doses of rapid-acting insulin to cover hyperglycemia and carbohydrate intake (ultimately using carbohydrate counting when feasible).

Carbohydrate estimation for breastfed infants can be challenging. If patients are fed pumped breastmilk, the carbohydrate content can be estimated at approximately 2.1 g per ounce of breastmilk. Resources are available to help caregivers estimate the quantity of breastmilk and, subsequently, the carbohydrates consumed.[46]

Continuous Subcutaneous Insulin Infusion Therapy

During the neonatal period, dosing can be difficult because of the frequent intake and variability in quantity. In addition, infants with neonatal diabetes are susceptible to hypoglycemia because of the relatively low insulin requirements.[47] Subcutaneous insulin infusions allow for very small accurate doses to be given in a physiologic way, with a continuous basal dose (as low as 0.025 units per hour) that may be adjusted hourly. In addition, pump technology allows for frequent hyperglycemia or carbohydrate bolus coverage (with doses typically as low as 0.05 units) while minimizing the potential for dangerous stacking of boluses.

All pediatric patients with diabetes (including neonatal diabetes) are candidates for CSII regardless of age.[48] Most observational studies have noted a decreased rate of hypoglycemic events, as well as reduced hemoglobin A_{1c}, in those receiving CSII rather than MDI.[44]

When deciding on the type of insulin pump to use, the following should be considered:

- Small basal rate increments allow for a lower hourly infusion rate; different varieties of insulin pumps may have the lowest setting of 0.025 units per hour versus 0.05 units per hour. It may also be important to consider using a pump that can be programmed to deliver no insulin (0.00 units per hour).
- Consider whether there is communication with a home glucose meter, whereby data collected from the glucometer is electronically communicated to the pump directly.
- Consider the types of infusion sets and tubing. For babies with less subcutaneous fat, infusion sets using a steel needle, or sets with a 30° insertion with a shorter cannula, may be more effective. Similar to older patients who have more lean mass and less fat, such catheters may be more effectively threaded into the subcutaneous tissue manually rather than using an inserter device. However, if using sites that have more fat, including the buttocks, a 90° insertion set may be used. One should consider that the buttocks may be a problematic site because of friction with clothing and diapers and exposure to stool. Of note, shorter tubing is generally preferred for small dose administration.
- Determine if there are alarm features.
- Waterproof casing in active children is important.

In general, assessment of capillary blood sugars in early infancy can be difficult because of the limited surface area and trauma-related concerns. Continuous glucose monitoring can be a very helpful tool for glucose control and parental reassurance, regardless of treatment modality. Studies with continuous glucose monitoring systems (CGMS) in very-low-birth-weight infants reveal a higher prevalence of abnormal glucose levels as compared with standard sampling methods. A study by Iglesias Platas and colleagues[49] showed no adverse events associated with CGMS and, with less associated fibrosis as compared with adults, sensors may be placed for longer periods of time in preterm infants. The thigh and upper buttock area in patients with little subcutaneous fat provide ideal insertion sites for insulin pumps and CGMs.[50]

Sulfonylureas

SU-responsive mutations are the most common cause of neonatal diabetes. Up to 90% to 95% of patients with NDM caused by *KCNJ11* may be successfully transitioned completely off of insulin therapy with a significant decrease in glycated hemoglobin levels.[19] In addition to the importance of the specific mutation, 2 large studies have also shown an association of improved and expedited response with initiation of therapy at an earlier age; this may result from impaired perinatal expansion or reduced replication of beta-cells with age.[51,52]

A significant proportion of patients exhibit a spectrum of neurodevelopmental disability related to the expression of mutated K-ATP channels in the brain, where SU therapy may also lead to beneficial effects on neurocognitive development.[53,54] Patients with *KCNJ11* mutations have reduced general intellectual ability, including reasoning, vocabulary, reading, and auditory working memory, as compared with sibling controls.[21] There is some evidence for improved neurocognitive outcomes with SU therapy, but the degree of benefit may depend on earlier age of treatment.[23,47]

A trial of glyburide may be considered in newly diagnosed neonatal diabetes because of the relatively high chance of having a mutation responsive to treatment (**Fig. 2**). In patients referred to the Monogenic Diabetes Registry, the authors found

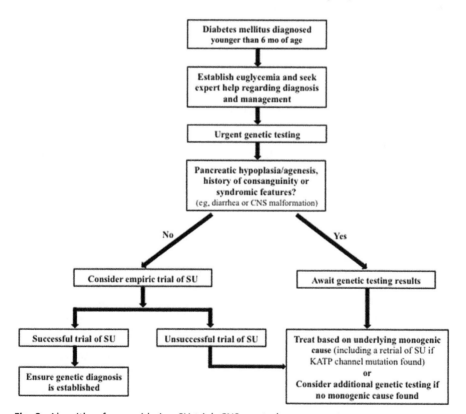

Fig. 2. Algorithm for considering SU trial. CNS, central nervous system.

that there was a mean delay of 10 weeks from the time of the diabetes diagnosis to the genetic diagnosis of NDM (range 1.6–58.2 weeks).[30] Because of the potential neurocognitive effects of delaying therapy, the authors, thus, suggest that a trial of SU therapy can be considered even before a genetic diagnosis is made, although genetic testing must be done in all cases. In patients with NDM who are responsive to SU therapy, glycemic outcomes are favorable and side effects are minimal.[19] There is some risk of hypoglycemia, although the risk seems to be much lower compared with insulin therapy.[30]

Approach to Transitioning from Insulin to Oral Glyburide

If patients are on CSII (pump), the basal rate should be reduced by 50% before glyburide administration.[19] The basal rate may be adjusted or suspended as needed to prevent hypoglycemia during transition. Glyburide tablets can be crushed and readily prepared in aqueous suspension; although the stability has not been well studied, the authors have not experienced any problems with the use of such a suspension for 14 days. An initial dosage of 0.1 mg per kilogram per dose twice daily before meals is most often used. The point-of-care BG should be assessed at least before a meal and at bedtime. On each subsequent day, if the BG is greater than 200 mg/dL at the time glyburide is due, the dose can be increased by 0.1 mg per kilogram per dose. The dose may, thus, be increased each day, progressing up to a dosage of at least 1 mg/kg/d (usually achieved within 5–7 days) if the premeal capillary blood sugars continue to be greater than 200 mg/dL.[30] If the patients' point of care glucose is less than 200 mg/dL, the usual prandial insulin dose should be reduced by at least 50%. In addition, doses of insulin should only be administered at least 2 to 3 hours after glyburide is dosed to avoid hypoglycemia. **Table 2** summarizes the authors' general approach to transition from insulin to oral glyburide therapy.

The original protocol[19] used a BG of 126 mg/dL as a threshold for dose titration. In the authors' experience it is often better to allow a reasonable level of hyperglycemia so as to avoid hypoglycemia while insulin is also being given, especially in neonates. Although it is very important to avoid extreme hyperglycemia, we have found 200 mg/dL to be a reasonable threshold for dose titration, but this may be altered based on specific clinical scenarios and the clinical judgment of the treating team.

Response to oral medications should be achieved in those with channel mutations including *KCNJ11* and *ABCC8*. However, some nonchannel mutations, such as 6q24, have been responsive to SU therapy as well.[31] If the desired effect is difficult to assess, glucose and C-peptide levels may be drawn before a meal and again 90 to 120 minutes after a meal is eaten (and glyburide is given). Patients with appropriate response to glyburide should have an appreciable increase in C-peptide level following glyburide dosing and a meal. If no clinical response or appreciable C-peptide difference is seen, then SU treatment should be discontinued and the patient managed on insulin therapy until genetic testing results are available.

Glyburide transition may also be done as an outpatient, depending on the families' comfort level with diabetes and insulin management. Once insulin has been completely discontinued, or a steady dose of glyburide has been achieved, patients should continue to monitor the BG levels before meals and at bedtime. Patients should also see their provider monthly for the first 6 months, followed by every 3 months thereafter.

Table 2
Transition from insulin to oral sulfonylurea therapy (specifically glyburide)

Day	Glucose Monitoring	Insulin Adjustments	Glyburide Dosing
Prep	Monitor the capillary BG before meals, 2 h after meals, bedtime, and 2 AM. Monitor the ketones when BG >300. Have a plan for hypoglycemia.	Maintain usual insulin regimen via pump or customary basal-bolus injections. Reduce the basal insulin by 50% (pump: decrease before breakfast on day 1; long-acting: reduce in the evening before transition)	Tablets available (may be halved) are as follows: 1.25, 2.5, or 5.0 mg. For infants, tablets may be crushed and suspended in formula or water.
1	Monitor the capillary BG before meals, bedtime, and 2 AM. If BG before a meal is >200 mg/dL (11.1 mmol/L) ↑↑ <200 mg/dL (11.1 mmol/L)	Administer rapid-acting bolus insulin as needed based on the capillary BG (unless glyburide is given within the last 2 h[a]): Give the usual bolus dose. Give 50% of the usual insulin dose.	Start with 0.1 mg/kg before breakfast and dinner (total 0.2 mg/kg/d). Depending on BG at the second dose, consider skipping a dose if BG is trending low.
2–7	Monitor the capillary BG before meals, bedtime, and 2 AM. If BG before SU dose is >200 mg/dL (11.1 mmol/L) ↑↑ <200 mg/dL (11.1 mmol/L)	Continue to wean down the basal dose as tolerated. Administer rapid-acting bolus insulin as needed based on the capillary BG: Give bolus dose from the previous day. Decrease the bolus dose by 50%.	Each day the dose will increase by 0.2 mg/kg/d (0.1 mg/kg per dose) depending on BGs. ↑ Increase the dose by 0.1 mg/kg. ↑ Continue the dose from the previous day.
Last	On the final day and after discharge, continue checking BG at least before every meal/feed, bedtime, and 2 AM to monitor the response. Relative hypoglycemia may necessitate lowering of the glyburide dose in the following weeks to months.	In most SU-responsive cases, insulin can be discontinued in 5–7 d, although mild hyperglycemia may occur. Treat with last titrated short-acting bolus insulin as needed. In some cases, low-dose basal insulin may be needed as well.	By the end of 5–7 d, patients will have either clearly responded to a lower dose or will be on at least 1 mg/kg/d. The dose may continue to be increased after discharge, with some patients requiring up to 2.0–2.5 mg/kg/d (which may be lowered in the following weeks to months).
Notes	If the expected response is uncertain, C-peptide levels before and after (90–120 min after) a meal and glyburide (no insulin) may be done, particularly when the dose is maximized at 1 mg/kg/d. If levels before SU are nearly undetectable but show a significant increment on glyburide, responsiveness is likely. Consider a further increase up to 2.0–2.5 mg/kg/d as needed.	BG ranges and insulin adjustments are only a guideline; the physician should be guided by clinical judgment. If there is any indication that glyburide is helping to control BG levels overall, it is often better to decrease the insulin aggressively so as to avoid hypoglycemia.	Patients with neurodevelopmental disability or those who are older at the time of transition may require higher doses of glyburide. In such cases, the possible benefit of continuing a high dose for the long-term should be carefully considered even if patients still require insulin.

[a] If glyburide was given in last 2 hours or with current BG check, recheck with next feed only; do not give insulin.

SUMMARY

NDM is caused by a single gene mutation. These patients will most often present within the first 6 months of life but, less commonly, may present at up to 12 months of life. Early clarification of the molecular cause by genetic testing is paramount. Patients with channel mutations, such as *KCNJ11* and *ABCC8,* can be transitioned to SU agents, allowing for simplified administration, decreased treatment costs, and potential neurodevelopmental improvements. Genetic testing may also guide longitudinal monitoring for other associated problems in forms with syndromic features as well as for screening of family members. Patients with 6q24 have a transient hyperglycemia in infancy with the onset of diabetes in adolescence. It is important to distinguish monogenic NDM from other causes of hyperglycemia in the newborn. Insulin-dependent hyperglycemia that persists longer than a week to 10 days, should raise suspicion for an underlying monogenic cause of diabetes and prompt genetic testing.

Best Practices

- There are more than 20 known monogenic causes of NDM, which may be transient or permanent (see **Table 1**).
- Genetic testing should be pursued in any infant with neonatal diabetes, even if hyperglycemia resolves. An underlying monogenic cause can lead to major differences in clinical management and is highly likely when diabetes is diagnosed at less than 6 months of age and less likely but still possible in infants with diabetes between 6 and 12 months of age.
- Hyperglycemia due to stress or illness may occur in neonates, especially in those who are premature or had very low birth weight (see **Fig. 2**). Diagnosis of diabetes (and genetic testing) should be considered:
  - Consider the diagnosis when hyperglycemia (glucose >250 mg/dL) persists beyond a few days without alternative explanation.
  - Consider the diagnosis when true serum glucose levels exceed 300 mg/dL, regardless of the time course.
  - Consider the diagnosis in any infant requiring insulin before 6 to 12 months of age.
- In neonates or infants, the authors would recommend using CSII to titrate insulin more precisely and better control blood sugar levels.
- SU responsive mutations are the most common causes of neonatal diabetes, and early treatment with SUs may improve neurocognitive deficits associated with these mutations. A trial of SU (glyburide) may be considered even before the genetic testing results are available (see **Fig. 2**).
- Depending on the age of patients and the comfort level of the families, transition insulin therapy to oral glyburide may be done as an inpatient or from home. See **Table 2** for guidance on medication transition.

REFERENCES

1. Letourneau LR, Carmody D, Wroblewski K, et al. Diabetes presentation in infancy: high risk of diabetic ketoacidosis. Diabetes Care 2017;40:e147–8.
2. De Franco E, Flanagan SE, Houghton JA, et al. The effect of early, comprehensive genomic testing on clinical care in neonatal diabetes: an international cohort study. Lancet 2015;386:957–63. Available at: http://linkinghub.elsevier.com/retrieve/pii/S0140673615600988. Accessed July 16, 2017.
3. Shah RP, Spruyt K, Kragie BC, et al. Visuomotor performance in KCNJ11-related neonatal diabetes is impaired in children with DEND-associated mutations and

may be improved by early treatment with sulfonylureas. Diabetes Care 2012;35: 2086–8. Available at: http://care.diabetesjournals.org/cgi/doi/10.2337/dc11-2225. Accessed July 16, 2017.

4. Hattersley A, Bruining J, Shield J, et al. ISPAD clinical practice consensus guidelines 2006-2007. The diagnosis and management of monogenic diabetes in children. Pediatr Diabetes 2006;7:352–60. Available at: http://doi.wiley.com/10.1111/j.1399-5448.2006.00217.x. Accessed July 16, 2017.

5. Besser REJ, Flanagan SE, Mackay DGJ, et al. Prematurity and genetic testing for neonatal diabetes. Pediatrics 2016;138:e20153926. Available at: http://pediatrics.aappublications.org/cgi/doi/10.1542/peds.2015-3926. Accessed July 16, 2017.

6. Beardsall K, Vanhaesebrouck S, Ogilvy-Stuart AL, et al. Prevalence and determinants of hyperglycemia in very low birth weight infants: cohort analyses of the NIRTURE study. J Pediatr 2010;157:715–9.e3. Available at: http://linkinghub.elsevier.com/retrieve/pii/S002234761000332X. Accessed July 16, 2017.

7. Sabzehei MK, Afjeh SA, Shakiba M, et al. Hyperglycemia in VLBW infants; incidence, risk factors and outcome. Arch Iran Med 2014;17:429–34.

8. Rozance PJ, Hay WW. Neonatal hyperglycemia. Neoreviews 2010;11:e632–9. Available at: http://neoreviews.aappublications.org/lookup/doi/10.1542/neo.11-11-e632. Accessed July 16, 2017.

9. Ogilvy-Stuart AL, Beardsall K. Management of hyperglycaemia in the preterm infant. Arch Dis Child Fetal Neonatal Ed 2010;95:F126–31. Available at: http://fn.bmj.com/cgi/doi/10.1136/adc.2008.154716. Accessed July 16, 2017.

10. Greeley SAW, Naylor RN, Philipson LH, et al. Neonatal diabetes: an expanding list of genes allows for improved diagnosis and treatment. Curr Diab Rep 2011;11:519–32. Available at: http://link.springer.com/10.1007/s11892-011-0234-7. Accessed July 16, 2017.

11. Naylor RN, Greeley SAW, Bell GI, et al. Genetics and pathophysiology of neonatal diabetes mellitus: neonatal diabetes mellitus. J Diabetes Investig 2011;2:158–69. Available at: http://doi.wiley.com/10.1111/j.2040-1124.2011.00106.x. Accessed July 16, 2017.

12. Ziegler AG, Hummel M, Schenker M, et al. Autoantibody appearance and risk for development of childhood diabetes in offspring of parents with type 1 diabetes: the 2-year analysis of the German BABYDIAB Study. Diabetes 1999;48:460–8. Available at: http://diabetes.diabetesjournals.org/cgi/doi/10.2337/diabetes.48.3.460. Accessed July 25, 2017.

13. Rubio-Cabezas O, Ellard S. Diabetes mellitus in neonates and infants: genetic heterogeneity, clinical approach to diagnosis, and therapeutic options. Horm Res Paediatr 2013;80:137–46. Available at: http://www.karger.com?doi=10.1159/000354219. Accessed July 16, 2017.

14. Karges B, Meissner T, Icks A, et al. Management of diabetes mellitus in infants. Nat Rev Endocrinol 2011;8:201–11. Available at: http://www.nature.com/doifinder/10.1038/nrendo.2011.204. Accessed July 16, 2017.

15. Patterson CC, Dahlquist GG, Gyürüs E, et al. Incidence trends for childhood type 1 diabetes in Europe during 1989–2003 and predicted new cases 2005–20: a multicentre prospective registration study. Lancet 2009;373:2027–33. Available at: http://linkinghub.elsevier.com/retrieve/pii/S0140673609605687. Accessed July 16, 2017.

16. Alkorta-Aranburu G, Sukhanova M, Carmody D, et al. Improved molecular diagnosis of patients with neonatal diabetes using a combined next-generation sequencing and MS-MLPA approach. J Pediatr Endocrinol Metab

2016;29:523–31. Available at: https://www.degruyter.com/view/j/jpem.2016.29. issue-5/jpem-2015-0341/jpem-2015-0341.xml. Accessed October 16, 2017.

17. Greeley SAW, John PM, Winn AN, et al. The cost-effectiveness of personalized genetic medicine: the case of genetic testing in neonatal diabetes. Diabetes Care 2011;34:622–7. Available at: http://care.diabetesjournals.org/cgi/doi/10. 2337/dc10-1616. Accessed July 16, 2017.

18. Rafiq M, Flanagan SE, Patch A-M, et al, The Neonatal Diabetes International Collaborative Group. Effective treatment with oral sulfonylureas in patients with diabetes due to sulfonylurea receptor 1 (SUR1) mutations. Diabetes Care 2008; 31:204–9. Available at: http://care.diabetesjournals.org/cgi/doi/10.2337/dc07-1785. Accessed July 16, 2017.

19. Pearson ER, Flechtner I, Njølstad PR, et al. Switching from insulin to oral sulfonyl-ureas in patients with diabetes due to Kir6.2 mutations. N Engl J Med 2006;355: 467–77. Available at: http://www.nejm.org/doi/abs/10.1056/NEJMoa061759. Accessed July 12, 2017.

20. Gloyn AL, Pearson ER, Antcliff JF, et al. Activating mutations in the gene encoding the ATP-sensitive potassium-channel subunit Kir6.2 and permanent neonatal diabetes. N Engl J Med 2004;350:1838–49. Available at: http://www.nejm.org/doi/abs/10.1056/NEJMoa032922. Accessed July 16, 2017.

21. Carmody D, Pastore AN, Landmeier KA, et al. Patients with *KCNJ11*-related diabetes frequently have neuropsychological impairments compared with sibling controls. Diabet Med 2016;33:1380–6. Available at: http://doi.wiley.com/10. 1111/dme.13159. Accessed July 16, 2017.

22. Landmeier KA, Lanning M, Carmody D, et al. ADHD, learning difficulties and sleep disturbances associated with *KCNJ11*-related neonatal diabetes. Pediatr Diabetes 2017;18(7):518–23. Available at: http://doi.wiley.com/10.1111/pedi. 12428. Accessed July 16, 2017.

23. Mohamadi A, Clark LM, Lipkin PH, et al. Medical and developmental impact of transition from subcutaneous insulin to oral glyburide in a 15-yr-old boy with neonatal diabetes mellitus and intermediate DEND syndrome: extending the age of KCNJ11 mutation testing in neonatal DM. Pediatr Diabetes 2009;11: 203–7. Available at: http://doi.wiley.com/10.1111/j.1399-5448.2009.00548.x. Accessed July 16, 2017.

24. Mlynarski W, Tarasov AI, Gach A, et al. Sulfonylurea improves CNS function in a case of intermediate DEND syndrome caused by a mutation in KCNJ11. Nat Clin Pract Neurol 2007;3:640–5. Available at: http://www.nature.com/doifinder/10. 1038/ncpneuro0640. Accessed July 16, 2017.

25. Slingerland AS, Nuboer R, Hadders-Algra M, et al. Improved motor development and good long-term glycaemic control with sulfonylurea treatment in a patient with the syndrome of intermediate developmental delay, early-onset generalised epilepsy and neonatal diabetes associated with the V59M mutation in the KCNJ11 gene. Diabetologia 2006;49:2559–63. Available at: http://link.springer. com/10.1007/s00125-006-0407-0. Accessed July 16, 2017.

26. Flanagan SE, Patch A-M, Mackay DJG, et al. Mutations in ATP-sensitive K+ channel genes cause transient neonatal diabetes and permanent diabetes in childhood or adulthood. Diabetes 2007;56:1930–7. Available at: http://diabetes. diabetesjournals.org/cgi/doi/10.2337/db07-0043. Accessed July 16, 2017.

27. Temple IK, Shield JPH. 6q24 transient neonatal diabetes. Rev Endocr Metab Disord 2010;11:199–204. Available at: http://link.springer.com/10.1007/s11154-010-9150-4. Accessed July 16, 2017.

28. Docherty LE, Kabwama S, Lehmann A, et al. Clinical presentation of 6q24 transient neonatal diabetes mellitus (6q24 TNDM) and genotype–phenotype correlation in an international cohort of patients. Diabetologia 2013;56:758–62. Available at: http://link.springer.com/10.1007/s00125-013-2832-1. Accessed July 16, 2017.

29. Flanagan SE, Mackay DJG, Greeley SAW, et al. Hypoglycaemia following diabetes remission in patients with 6q24 methylation defects: expanding the clinical phenotype. Diabetologia 2013;56:218–21. Available at: http://link.springer.com/10.1007/s00125-012-2766-z. Accessed July 16, 2017.

30. Carmody D, Bell CD, Hwang JL, et al. Sulfonylurea treatment before genetic testing in neonatal diabetes: pros and cons. J Clin Endocrinol Metab 2014;99: E2709–14. Available at: https://academic.oup.com/jcem/article-lookup/doi/10.1210/jc.2014-2494. Accessed July 12, 2017.

31. Carmody D, Beca FA, Bell CD, et al. Role of noninsulin therapies alone or in combination in chromosome 6q24-related transient neonatal diabetes: sulfonylurea improves but does not always normalize insulin secretion: table 1. Diabetes Care 2015;38:e86–7. Available at: http://care.diabetesjournals.org/lookup/doi/10.2337/dc14-3056. Accessed July 16, 2017.

32. Yorifuji T, Hashimoto Y, Kawakita R, et al. Relapsing 6q24-related transient neonatal diabetes mellitus successfully treated with a dipeptidyl peptidase-4 inhibitor: a case report. Pediatr Diabetes 2014;15:606–10. Available at: http://doi.wiley.com/10.1111/pedi.12123. Accessed July 16, 2017.

33. Edghill EL, Flanagan SE, Patch A-M, et al. Insulin mutation screening in 1,044 patients with diabetes: mutations in the INS gene are a common cause of neonatal diabetes but a rare cause of diabetes diagnosed in childhood or adulthood. Diabetes 2008;57:1034–42. Available at: http://diabetes.diabetesjournals.org/cgi/doi/10.2337/db07-1405. Accessed July 24, 2017.

34. Liu M, Hodish I, Haataja L, et al. Proinsulin misfolding and diabetes: mutant INS gene-induced diabetes of youth. Trends Endocrinol Metab 2010;21:652–9. Available at: http://linkinghub.elsevier.com/retrieve/pii/S1043276010001219. Accessed October 14, 2017.

35. Park S-Y, Ye H, Steiner DF, et al. Mutant proinsulin proteins associated with neonatal diabetes are retained in the endoplasmic reticulum and not efficiently secreted. Biochem Biophys Res Commun 2010;391:1449–54. Available at: http://linkinghub.elsevier.com/retrieve/pii/S0006291X09024632. Accessed July 16, 2017.

36. Støy J, Steiner DF, Park S-Y, et al. Clinical and molecular genetics of neonatal diabetes due to mutations in the insulin gene. Rev Endocr Metab Disord 2010;11: 205–15. Available at: http://link.springer.com/10.1007/s11154-010-9151-3. Accessed July 16, 2017.

37. De Franco E, Shaw-Smith C, Flanagan SE, et al. GATA6 mutations cause a broad phenotypic spectrum of diabetes from pancreatic agenesis to adult-onset diabetes without exocrine insufficiency. Diabetes 2013;62:993–7. Available at: http://diabetes.diabetesjournals.org/cgi/doi/10.2337/db12-0885. Accessed July 16, 2017.

38. Delépine M, Nicolino M, Barrett T, et al. EIF2AK3, encoding translation initiation factor 2-alpha kinase 3, is mutated in patients with Wolcott-Rallison syndrome. Nat Genet 2000;25:406–9.

39. Bennett CL, Christie J, Ramsdell F, et al. The immune dysregulation, polyendocrinopathy, enteropathy, X-linked syndrome (IPEX) is caused by mutations of FOXP3. Nat Genet 2001;27:20–1.

40. Patel KA, Oram RA, Flanagan SE, et al. Type 1 diabetes genetic risk score: a novel tool to discriminate monogenic and type 1 diabetes. Diabetes 2016;65: 2094–9. Available at: http://diabetes.diabetesjournals.org/lookup/doi/10.2337/db15-1690. Accessed July 24, 2017.

41. Bottino M, Cowett RM, Sinclair JC. Interventions for treatment of neonatal hyperglycemia in very low birth weight infants. In: The Cochrane Collaboration, editor. Cochrane database of systematic reviews. Chichester (United Kingdom): John Wiley & Sons, Ltd; 2011. Available at: http://doi.wiley.com/10.1002/14651858. CD007453.pub3. Accessed July 24, 2017.

42. Humalog [package insert]. Eli Lilly and Company; 1996. Available at: http://pi.lilly.com/us/humalog-pen-pi.pdf. Accessed November 28, 2017.

43. Novolog [package insert]. Novo Nordisk; 2017. Available at: http://www.novo-pi.com/novolog.pdf. Accessed November 28, 2017.

44. Phillip M, Battelino T, Rodriguez H, et al, for the Consensus forum participants. Use of insulin pump therapy in the pediatric age-group: consensus statement from the European Society for Paediatric Endocrinology, the Lawson Wilkins Pediatric Endocrine Society, and the International Society for Pediatric and Adolescent Diabetes, endorsed by the American Diabetes Association and the European Association for the Study of Diabetes. Diabetes Care 2007;30: 1653–62. Available at: http://care.diabetesjournals.org/cgi/doi/10.2337/dc07-9922. Accessed July 16, 2017.

45. Danne T, Bangstad H-J, Deeb L, et al. Insulin treatment in children and adolescents with diabetes: insulin treatment. Pediatr Diabetes 2014;15:115–34. Available at: http://doi.wiley.com/10.1111/pedi.12184. Accessed October 16, 2017.

46. Miller D, Mamilly L, Fourtner S, et al, the Academy of Breastfeeding Medicine. ABM clinical protocol #27: breastfeeding an infant or young child with insulin-dependent diabetes. Breastfeed Med 2017;12:72–6. Available at: http://online.liebertpub.com/doi/10.1089/bfm.2017.29035.djm. Accessed July 16, 2017.

47. Bharucha T, Brown J, McDonnell C, et al. Neonatal diabetes mellitus: insulin pump as an alternative management strategy. J Paediatr Child Health 2005;41: 522–6. Available at: http://doi.wiley.com/10.1111/j.1440-1754.2005.00696.x. Accessed July 16, 2017.

48. Kapellen TM, Heidtmann B, Lilienthal E, et al, for the DPV-Science-Initiative, the German Working Group for Pediatric Pump Treatment, the German Competence Network Diabetes. Continuous subcutaneous insulin infusion in neonates and infants below 1 year: analysis of initial bolus and basal rate based on the experiences from the German working group for pediatric pump treatment. Diabetes Technol Ther 2015;17:872–9. Available at: http://online.liebertpub.com/doi/10.1089/dia.2015.0030. Accessed October 17, 2017.

49. Iglesias Platas I, Thió Lluch M, Pociello Almiñana N, et al. Continuous glucose monitoring in infants of very low birth weight. Neonatology 2009;95:217–23. Available at: http://www.karger.com/doi/10.1159/000165980. Accessed July 16, 2017.

50. Beardsall K, Vanhaesebrouck S, Ogilvy-Stuart AL, et al. Early insulin therapy in very-low-birth-weight infants. N Engl J Med 2008;359:1873–84. Available at: http://www.nejm.org/doi/abs/10.1056/NEJMoa0803725. Accessed July 16, 2017.

51. The United States Neonatal Diabetes Working Group, Thurber BW, Carmody D, Tadie EC, et al. Age at the time of sulfonylurea initiation influences treatment outcomes in KCNJ11-related neonatal diabetes. Diabetologia 2015;58:1430–5. Available at: http://link.springer.com/10.1007/s00125-015-3593-9. Accessed July 16, 2017.

52. Babiker T, Vedovato N, Patel K, et al. Successful transfer to sulfonylureas in KCNJ11 neonatal diabetes is determined by the mutation and duration of diabetes. Diabetologia 2016;59:1162–6. Available at: http://link.springer.com/10.1007/s00125-016-3921-8. Accessed October 17, 2017.

53. Fujimura N, Tanaka E, Yamamoto S, et al. Contribution of ATP-sensitive potassium channels to hypoxic hyperpolarization in rat hippocampal CA1 neurons in vitro. J Neurophysiol 1997;77:378–85.

54. Beltrand J, Elie C, Busiah K, et al. Sulfonylurea therapy benefits neurological and psychomotor functions in patients with neonatal diabetes owing to potassium channel mutations. Diabetes Care 2015;38:2033–41. Available at: http://care.diabetesjournals.org/lookup/doi/10.2337/dc15-0837. Accessed July 24, 2017.

Hyperinsulinism in the Neonate

Katherine Lord, MD[a,b], Diva D. De León, MD, MSCE[a,b],*

KEYWORDS

- Hypoglycemia • Neonate • Hyperinsulinism • Insulin • Pancreas • Pancreatectomy

KEY POINTS

- Hyperinsulinism (HI) is the most common cause of persistent hypoglycemia and is associated with high rates of neurodevelopmental deficits.
- Prompt evaluation to establish the diagnosis is important to start appropriate treatment.
- As soon as a diagnosis of HI is established, an initial trial of diazoxide is necessary to identify those who are likely to benefit from specialized evaluation.
- Infants with diazoxide-unresponsive HI require expedited genetic testing for *ABCC8* and *KCNJ11* to determine the likelihood of focal disease.
- The goal of medical therapy is to allow infants to maintain normal feeding patterns and to sustain plasma glucose greater than 70 mg/dL.

INTRODUCTION

Hyperinsulinism (HI), the most common cause of persistent hypoglycemia in infants, carries a high risk of long-term morbidity. In HI, dysregulated insulin secretion results in severe hypoglycemia, suppression of the counterregulatory response to hypoglycemia, and, more significantly, suppression of ketone bodies production, which are crucial alternative fuels for the brain. Thus, severe and recurrent hypoketotic hypoglycemia resulting from HI, if untreated, is associated with irreversible brain damage. The frequency of neurodevelopmental delays in HI is as high as 30% to 50% and, importantly, this affects not only children with congenital and permanent forms of HI but also children with transient HI.[1–3] Prompt recognition and appropriate management are critical to decrease the risk of these poor outcomes. Elucidation of the molecular genetics of HI and advances in diagnostic testing, specifically the use of 18-fluoro-L-3,4-dihydroxyphenylalanine (^{18}F-DOPA) PET to localize focal lesions, has resulted in a personalized approach to management and decreased morbidity.

Disclosure Statement: The authors have nothing to disclose.
[a] The Division of Endocrinology and Diabetes, The Children's Hospital of Philadelphia, 3401 Civic Center Boulevard, Philadelphia, PA 19104, USA; [b] Department of Pediatrics, The Perelman School of Medicine, University of Pennsylvania, 3401 Civic Center Boulevard, Philadelphia, PA 19104, USA
* Corresponding author. The Children's Hospital of Philadelphia, Abramson Research Center, Room 802A, 3615 Civic Center Boulevard, Philadelphia, PA.
E-mail address: deleon@email.chop.edu

EPIDEMIOLOGY

The incidence of congenital HI is approximately 1 in 50,000 live births.[4] In addition to the monogenic forms of congenital HI, HI can be transient and related to perinatal stress or may be part of an underlying syndrome (**Box 1**).[5,6]

Perinatal Stress-Induced Hyperinsulinism

It is well established that plasma glucose concentrations are lower in the first 1 day to 3 days of life in normal newborns, a period of transitional glucose regulation that may be explained by a lower plasma glucose threshold for suppression of insulin secretion.[7] The process of β-cell maturation after birth may be impacted by perinatal factors, resulting in perinatal stress-induced HI, which can be common in these at-risk neonates. In a study of 514 neonates at risk of hypoglycemia, 47% of late-preterm and small-for-gestational-age (SGA) infants were found to have hypoglycemia during the first 48 hours of life[8]; 19% of the babies had recurrent episodes. A majority of infants with perinatal stress HI are diazoxide-responsive, although a subset, in particular those with hypoxic ischemic encephalopathy and liver dysfunction, may fail to respond. Perinatal stress HI resolves within the first 3 months to 6 months of life.[6]

Box 1
Causes of hyperinsulinism

Congenital

- K_{ATP}-HI (*ABCC8, KCNJ11*)
- GDH-HI (*GLUD1*)
- GCK-HI (*GCK*)
- HNF4α-HI (*HNF4A*)
- HNF1α-HI (*HNF1A*)
- SCHAD-HI (*HADH*)
- UCP2-HI (*UCP2*)
- Exercise-induced HI (*SLC16A1*)
- Phosphoglucomutase 1 deficiency (*PGM1*)

Perinatal stress

- Intrauterine growth restriction
- Birth asphyxia
- Maternal preeclampsia/eclampsia
- Congenital heart disease
- Meconium aspiration syndrome
- Prematurity

Syndromic

- Beckwith-Wiedemann
- Turner
- Soto
- Kabuki

These neonates may be at risk for long-term neurologic deficits, however, as demonstrated by the study of a large cohort of neonates at risk followed-up to 4.5 years and found to have a dose-dependent increased risk of poor executive function and visual motor function.[9] Thus, identification and appropriate treatment of these neonates are important to prevent long-term neurologic deficits.

GENETICS

Abnormalities in 10 genes encoding proteins that play an important role in the regulation of insulin secretion are associated with HI (**Fig. 1**). The most common types are discussed.

ATP-Sensitive Potassium Channels–Hyperinsulinism

Inactivating mutations of *ABCC8* and *KCNJ11* that encode SUR1 and Kir6.2, the 2 components of the β-cell ATP-sensitive potassium (K_{ATP}) channels, cause the most common and severe form of congenital HI.[10,11] The mutations result in either lack of channels on the β-cell plasma membrane or channels that are expressed but have impaired function. These channel abnormalities lead to dysregulated insulin secretion, which in a majority of cases is unresponsive to diazoxide, a K_{ATP} channel agonist. Depending on the

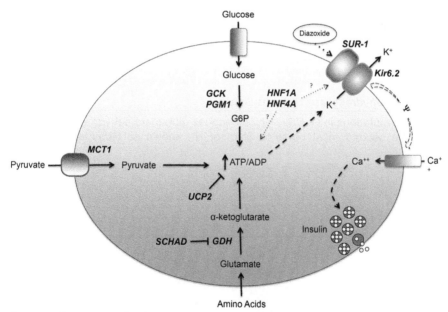

Fig. 1. Insulin secretion by the β cell and site of genetic defects causing HI. Glucose and amino acids are the major fuel signals in the β cell. ATP production from fuel metabolism results in closure of the K_{ATP} channel, which is composed of 2 subunits: SUR-1 and Kir6.2. Closure of the channel results in depolarization of the β cell membrane. The depolarization triggers opening of the voltage-sensitive calcium channels and the subsequent calcium influx leads to insulin secretion. Genetic defects (*bold italics*) in these pathways result in HI. Six are inactivating mutations: SUR-1 (sulfonylurea receptor 1), Kir6.2 (potassium channel), UCP2 (uncoupling protein 2), HNF4A, HNF1A, and SCHAD (short-chain 3-OH acyl-CoA dehydrogenase functioning as inhibitor of GDH through direct protein/protein interaction). Three are activating mutations: GCK, GDH, PGM1 (phosphoglucomutase 1), and MCT1 (monocarboxylate transporter 1). G6P, glucose-6-phosphate.

mutation and its impact on the channel expression and function, K_{ATP}-HI can be recessive diazoxide-unresponsive, dominant diazoxide-unresponsive, or dominant diazoxide-responsive.[12] Infants with diazoxide-unresponsive K_{ATP}-HI present with severe hypoglycemia, large-for-gestational-age (LGA) birth weight, and high glucose infusion rate (GIR) requirements. Infants with the diazoxide-responsive form typically present with milder disease.[13]

K_{ATP}-HI has 2 distinct histologic subtypes: diffuse and focal (**Fig. 2**). In diffuse K_{ATP}-HI, β-cells throughout the pancreas show signs of hyperactivity.[14] In contrast, a discrete area of β-cell proliferation or adenomatosis characterizes the focal form. Diffuse K_{ATP}-HI results from biallelic recessive mutations in the K_{ATP} genes; less commonly, dominant mutations are found. Focal K_{ATP}-HI is the result of a 2-hit mechanism: (1) a paternally inherited recessive mutation in *ABCC8* or *KCNJ11* and (2) somatic loss of the maternally inherited 11p15 chromosomal region, compensated by paternal uniparental disomy.[15,16] The histologic differences in the 2 forms lead to divergent treatment options and outcomes. Patients with focal K_{ATP}-HI are cured with resection of the focal lesion, whereas pancreatectomy for patients with the diffuse form is palliative.

Given these different outcomes, distinguishing between the focal and diffuse forms of K_{ATP}-HI is crucial. Neonates with the diffuse form are more likely to present at birth, whereas those with focal form may fail detection in the neonatal period and present at several weeks to months of life with hypoglycemia seizures.[17] Due to significant overlap in clinical presentation, however, clinical features alone cannot be used to distinguish between the 2 forms. Genetic testing offers the best means of identifying infants with focal K_{ATP}-HI: a single recessive paternally inherited mutation in *ABCC8* or *KCNJ11* has a positive predictive value of 94% for focal HI.[18]

Glutamate Dehydrogenase–Hyperinsulinism

Activating mutations in *GLUD1*, which encodes glutamate dehydrogenase (GDH), cause the second most common form of HI, known as HI/hyperammonemia

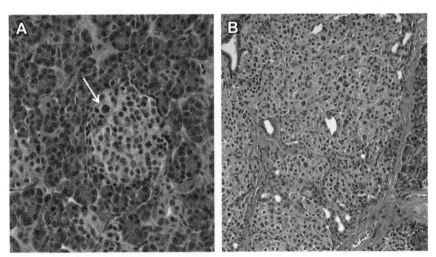

Fig. 2. (*A*) Section of pancreas from a diffuse case showing a pancreatic islet demonstrating β-cell nucleomegaly (*white arrow*), histologic hallmark of diffuse disease (H&E, original magnification × 400). (*B*) Adenomatous lesion from a case of focal HI (H&E, original magnification × 200). Normal pancreas tissue is seen on the right side of the image.

(HI/HA) syndrome.[19] GDH is involved in amino acid–stimulated insulin secretion. Mutations in *GLUD1* most commonly occur de novo (70%), with the remainder inherited in an autosomal dominant manner. Infants with HI/HA syndrome present with fasting and protein-induced hypoglycemia and ammonia levels 3 times to 5 times above the normal range. This form of HI is associated with increased rates of seizures and learning disabilities that may not be directly the result of the hypoglycemia or the HA.[20] Individuals with HI/HA syndrome are responsive to diazoxide.

Glucokinase-Hyperinsulinism

Glucokinase (GCK) is the key enzyme regulating the glucose threshold for insulin secretion.[21] Activating mutations of GCK, encoded by *GCK*, cause an autosomal dominant form of HI, which has variable degrees of severity and diazoxide responsiveness. Although most infants may be managed medically, the severe cases may require near-total pancreatectomy.[22]

Hepatic Nuclear Factor 4 Alpha—Hyperinsulinism

Mutations in the pancreatic transcription factor, hepatic nuclear factor 4 alpha (HNF4α), cause diazoxide-responsive HI.[23] Infants with HNF4A-HI are typically macrosomic and can be treated with low dose diazoxide. The hypoglycemia resolves within the first several years of life. Progressive β-cell failure occurs, however, and results in a monogenic form of early onset diabetes (maturity-onset diabetes of the young [MODY1]).[24] A similar clinical progression (from HI to diabetes) has been described in individuals with mutations in another pancreatic transcription factor, hepatic nuclear factor 1nalpha (HNF1α), which results in MODY3.[25]

DIAGNOSIS
Clinical Presentation

The classic presentation of HI is an LGA infant with a high GIR (>10 mg/kg/min), as is commonly seen in K_{ATP}-HI. The clinical phenotype, however, is a spectrum and some patients present with normal birth weight and minimally elevated glucose requirements. Clinical features can suggest a specific phenotype and guide genetic testing **(Box 2)**.

Indications for a Hypoglycemia Evaluation

An expert committee of pediatric endocrinologists and neonatologists recently published guidelines for the evaluation and management of hypoglycemia in neonates, infants, and children.[26] The committee recommended evaluation for a persistent hypoglycemia disorder in neonates unable to consistently maintain plasma glucose concentrations greater than 60 mg/dL by the third day of life, those with severe hypoglycemia (symptomatic hypoglycemia or requiring intravenous dextrose), and those who are at high risk of having a persistent hypoglycemic disorder (LGA, SGA, perinatal stress, maternal diabetes, congenital syndromes, or family history of genetic hypoglycemia disorders).

Laboratory Evaluation

A diagnosis of HI is based on a critical blood sample obtained at the time of hypoglycemia. The critical sample is used to measure plasma concentrations of the hormones and alternative fuels involved in the physiologic response to fasting. To minimize false-positive results, the plasma glucose threshold for obtaining a critical sample is less than 50 mg/dL. This sample may be obtained during a spontaneous episode of

---

Box 2
Clinical features of hyperinsulinism

High GIR (>10 mg/kg/min)
- All forms
- Highest in K_{ATP}-HI

LGA
- K_{ATP}-HI
- GCK-HI
- HNF4α and HNF1α-HI
- Beckwith-Wiedemann
- Soto

SGA
- Perinatal stress HI

Congenital heart disease
- Perinatal stress HI
- Turner
- Kabuki

Hypertrophic cardiomyopathy
- K_{ATP}-HI

---

hypoglycemia or during a carefully monitored fast. It is important to confirm the plasma glucose using a laboratory-based assay rather than relying on a point-of-care glucose. In addition to obtaining the critical sample, the glycemic response to glucagon should be assessed.[27] At the time of hypoglycemia (after obtaining the critical blood sample), 1 mg of glucagon is administered and plasma glucoses are monitored every 10 minutes for a total of 40 minutes. For practical reasons, typically, point-of-care meters are used for the measurements of plasma glucose after glucagon is administered. In HI, glucagon administration results in an increase of plasma glucose by greater than 30 mg/dL (**Box 3**). If the plasma glucose does not increase by 20 mg/dL in the first 20 minutes, however, the test should end and the infant should be fed.

The laboratory findings of HI include detectable insulin/C-peptide, suppressed β-hydroxybutyrate and free fatty acids, and an inappropriate glycemic response to glucagon (see **Box 3**). Insulin may not be detectable in a sample taken from peripheral blood (because of hepatic metabolism and/or a hemolyzed sample), so other evidence of insulin actions during hypoglycemia, such as suppression of lipolysis (suppressed free fatty acids), ketogenesis (suppressed β-hydroxybutyrate), and glycogenolysis (glycemic response to glucagon), must be used. Neonatal panhypopituitarism can have an identical biochemical profile to HI. If cortisol and growth hormone levels from the critical sample are not elevated, the appropriate stimulation tests should be performed to evaluate for possible hypopituitarism.[28]

Genetic Testing

Genetic testing should be considered in all patients diagnosed with HI and is available commercially for the known HI genes. By identifying a specific genotype,

---

Box 3
Diagnostic criteria

When plasma glucose less than 50 mg/dL

- Low β-hydroxybutyrate (<1.8 mmol/L)
- Low free fatty acids (<1.7 mmol)
- Plus/minus detectable insulin/C-peptide
- Positive glycemic response to glucagon (30-point rise in glucose)

Exclude neonatal panhypopituitarism:

- Cortisol greater than 10 μg/dL
- Growth hormone greater than 7 ng/mL

---

families can be counseled regarding comorbidities and expected duration of treatment, and the genotype result can aid in future family planning. Any infant who fails to respond to diazoxide should have expedited testing (4-day to 7-day turnaround time) of *ABCC8* and *KCNJ11*, because this suggests K_{ATP}-HI. If a mutation in *ABCC8* or *KCNJ11* is found, genotyping the parents is critical to determine parent-of-origin of the mutation and assess the likelihood of focal HI. Rapid identification of infants with the focal form allows the infants to more quickly undergo ^{18}F-DOPA PET and curative surgery.

MANAGEMENT

The goal of treatment in HI is to maintain plasma glucose greater than 70 mg/dL, even during periods of fasting. This goal is initially accomplished using dextrose-containing intravenous fluids. If central venous access is obtained, higher concentration dextrose can be used to minimize fluid overload. Throughout treatment, neonates and infants should be allowed to feed on demand. Nutritional modifications (fortified feedings and continuous feedings) alone are not sufficient to treat HI, and forced feedings or continuous feeds lead to oral aversion and poor feeding skills.

Medical Therapy

There are few medical treatment options for HI, which makes treatment challenging (**Table 1**). The mainstay of therapy is diazoxide, which opens the K_{ATP} channel on the β cell, resulting in inhibition of insulin secretion.[29,30] Side effects of diazoxide include fluid retention; thus, neonates and infants on diazoxide therapy require concomitant therapy with a diuretic, such as chlorothiazide. Diuretic use decreases the risk of fluid overload and respiration compromise, which is frequently seen with neonates receiving diazoxide and large amounts of intravenous fluids.

Octreotide, a somatostatin analog, is the second-line agent used in the treatment of HI.[31] Treatment failure is common, however, due to development of tachyphylaxis. Additionally, safety concerns have significantly limited its use in neonates. Octreotide has been associated with fatal necrotizing enterocolitis and should be avoided during the first 6 weeks to 8 weeks of life.[32,33] A long-acting somatostatin analogue, lanreotide, has been used successfully in children with HI, although dosing limitations restricts its use in the younger patients.[34,35] Finally, glucagon can be used as a continuous intravenous infusion of 1 mg per day to lower dextrose

Table 1
Medications for the treatment of hyperinsulinism in neonates and infants

Name	Dose	Route	Side Effects
Diazoxide	5–15 mg/kg/d, divided twice daily	Oral	Hypertrichosis, fluid retention, bone marrow suppression, decreased appetite
Chlorothiazide (concomitant use in children treated with diazoxide to avoid fluid retention)	20–40 mg/kg/d, divided twice daily	Oral	Hypokalemia
Octreotide	2–20 μg/kg/d, every 6–8 h	Subcutaneous	Elevated liver enzymes, diarrhea, gallstones, growth failure, hypothyroidism, necrotizing enterocolitis
Glucagon	1 mg/d, continuous infusion	Intavenos	Emesis, rash

needs in infants awaiting surgery. Solubility issues have limited its use in the outpatient setting.

Steroids are not effective therapy for HI and expose infants to unnecessary side effects, such as iatrogenic adrenal insufficiency, hypertension, and bone demineralization. Calcium channel blockers, such as nifedipine, also have limited effectiveness in this population and should not be used for treatment of HI.[36] In 2014, sirolimus, a mammalian target of rapamycin inhibitor, was reported as a novel treatment, but subsequent studies have failed to show efficacy.[37,38] Given the risks of increased susceptibility to severe infections associated with sirolimus, its use is not currently recommended.[39]

Assessing Diazoxide Responsiveness

After establishing the diagnosis of HI, a therapeutic trial of diazoxide to determine responsiveness is the crucial first step. Diazoxide is initiated at 5 mg/kg/d to 10 mg/kg/d (or higher in more severe cases) and if there is no improvement in plasma glucose after several days, titrated up to a maximum dose of 15 mg/kg/d. After 5 days on a stable dose of diazoxide, a 12-hour safety fast should be performed to assess responsiveness. Neonates are considered diazoxide-unresponsive if, after 5 days on the maximum dose, they continue to require dextrose support or are unable to maintain plasma glucoses greater than 70 mg/dL while fasting. At that time, the diazoxide should be discontinued and, as discussed previously, expedited genetic testing for *ABCC8* and *KCNJ11* should be sent, because mutations in 1 of these 2 genes account for greater than 90% of cases. These patients require referral to a specialized HI center as possible surgical candidates.

For children with diazoxide-unresponsive diffuse HI, medical therapy can be attempted with continuous enteral dextrose and after the neonatal period, octreotide. In those with severe disease, this approach may be insufficient due to limits on the amount of enteral dextrose that can be safely used as well as side effects from high doses of octreotide. These patients are often referred for surgical intervention. The risks and benefits of the 2 approaches are discussed in more detail later.

18-Fluoro-L-3,4-dihydroxyphenylalanine PET

The recognition that some patients with severe HI were cured after a partial pancreatectomy led to the identification of focal K_{ATP}-HI in the 1980s. Identifying patients with focal HI and accurately localizing the lesion in the pancreas became 2 of the biggest management challenges for the disease. Understanding the genetic mechanisms of HI led to the recognition that patients with focal HI carry paternally inherited *ABCC8* or *KCNJ11* mutations. Localization of the focal lesion, however, remained a challenge. Conventional imaging, such as ultrasound, CT, and MRI, cannot identify focal lesions, and interventional radiology techniques, such as arterial stimulation venous sampling, were invasive and had poor accuracy at localizing lesions.[40]

The introduction of the ^{18}F-DOPA PET scan was one of the most significant advances in the care of children with HI. Introduced in 2003, it is used to differentiate focal from diffuse disease and to localize focal lesions in the pancreas.[41,42] The tracer, ^{18}F-DOPA, is taken up by neuroendocrine tissue. In focal disease, there is an area of increased tracer uptake in a specific region of the pancreas, corresponding to the area of β-cell adenomatosis **(Fig. 3)**. In patients with diffuse HI, the uptake of tracer is uniform throughout the pancreas. In the largest published series to date, 105 infants with HI underwent ^{18}F-DOPA scans, followed by surgery.[43] The sensitivity and specificity for diagnosing focal disease were 85% and 96%, respectively; 100% of lesions were correctly localized in the pancreas.

All infants who have genetics consistent with focal HI require an ^{18}F-DOPA PET scan prior to surgery. Additionally, patients with diazoxide-unresponsive, genetic-negative HI should also undergo an ^{18}F-DOPA PET scan, because they still have the possibility of a focal lesion. Patients who are diazoxide-responsive or those with genetic results known to cause diffuse disease, such as biallelic recessive mutations in *ABCC8* or *KCNJ11* or a *GCK* mutation, do not benefit from imaging.

Surgical Intervention

Surgery is indicated for infants who have a focal lesion or those with diffuse disease who fail medical therapy. Patients with focal lesions should undergo surgery at

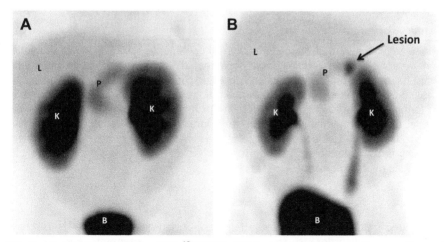

Fig. 3. (*A*) Frontal view of a MIP ^{18}F-DOPA PET image showing a uniform pattern of uptake throughout the pancreas, consistent with diffuse disease. (*B*) Frontal view of a MIP ^{18}F-DOPA PET image demonstrating increased uptake in the tail of the pancreas, consistent with a focal lesion (*black arrow*). Normal liver (L), kidney (K), pancreas (P), and bladder (B) uptake is seen in both images. MIP, maximum intensity projection.

specialized HI centers, which have the multidisciplinary expertise to ensure complete incision of the lesion while minimizing the amount of pancreas resected.[44] At the time of surgery, intraoperative ultrasound can be used to confirm the location of the focal lesion. Frozen section evaluation of biopsies by experienced pathologists allows for confirmation of the focal lesion and guides the extent of pancreatic resection.

Infants with diffuse HI requiring surgical intervention undergo near-total pancreatectomy with gastrostomy tube placement. The gastrostomy tube is necessary for postoperative management because a majority of patients continue to have hypoglycemia, although less severe.[17] For children with diffuse disease, the decision to proceed with surgery is complex and requires careful consideration of the risks and benefits. Surgery decreases the severity of the hypoglycemia and makes it easier to manage medically. This must be weighed, however, against the risk of a surgical procedure as well as the long-term complications of diabetes and pancreatic insufficiency. Medical therapy avoids these complications but carries its own risks with more exposure to hypoglycemia as well as side effects from the high doses of somatostatin analogs that are required.

PROGNOSIS
Surgical Outcomes

A review of 223 surgical cases from the Children's Hospital of Philadelphia found that 94% of infants with focal HI were cured and the majority required less than a 50% pancreatectomy.[17] In contrast, only a quarter of patients with diffuse disease were euglycemic after pancreatectomy. More than 40% of patients required continued treatment of hypoglycemia, and the remainder were treated for hyperglycemia.

Individuals who undergo near-total pancreatectomy in infancy have a high risk of developing diabetes.[2,45] More than 90% of these patients develop insulin-dependent diabetes mellitus during the first 2 decades of life; the median age at diagnosis of diabetes is 8 years.

Neurodevelopmental Outcomes

Despite advances in the field, children with HI continue to have a high risk of neurocognitive abnormalities. Studies have shown that 26% to 48% of children and adults with HI have developmental delays and neurologic issues and 13% to 25% have seizures.[1,46] Poor developmental outcomes are not only limited to children with persistent forms of HI but also involve children with transient forms of HI.[3] Furthermore, the rates of developmental delay and seizures for children treated in the 2000s remain similar to those individuals treated in the decades before.[2] These findings suggest the need for improved screening protocols to identify infants with HI as early as possible to avoid these neurologic sequela.

SUMMARY

With limited medical therapies and a high risk of neurologic damage, HI remains a challenging disorder to treat. Advances in management, such as the ^{18}F-DOPA PET scan, however, have resulted in improved outcomes for the subset of infants with focal HI. Ongoing research into the genetic and molecular basis of HI will hopefully result in novel treatments that benefit those infants with diffuse HI.

Best Practices

What is the current best practice?

- Prompt evaluation of infants with suspected HI
- Early identification of infants with focal K_{ATP}-HI and referral to specialized HI center for ^{18}F-DOPA PET

What changes in current practice are likely to improve outcomes?

- Support plasma glucose with intravenous fluids and allow infants to feed orally on demand
- Use of diuretics in all infants on diazoxide

Major recommendations

- Diagnostic evaluation of neonates who are at high risk of having a persistent hypoglycemic disorder
- Initiate trial of diazoxide as soon as diagnosis of HI is made
- Infants who are diazoxide-unresponsive require expedited genetic testing for *ABCC8* and *KCNJ11*
- The goal of medical therapy is to allow infants with HI to maintain plasma glucose greater than 70 mg/dL while fasting

Summary statement

Early recognition and appropriate treatment of infants with HI are crucial to avoid long-term complications, such as developmental delays and diabetes

---

ACKNOWLEDGMENTS

The authors thank Dr Trisha Bhatti for providing the histology images and Dr Lisa States for providing the ^{18}F-DOPA PET scan images.

REFERENCES

1. Meissner T, Wendel U, Burgard P, et al. Long-term follow-up of 114 patients with congenital hyperinsulinism. Eur J Endocrinol 2003;149(1):43–51.
2. Lord K, Radcliffe J, Gallagher PR, et al. High risk of diabetes and neurobehavioral deficits in individuals with surgically treated hyperinsulinism. J Clin Endocrinol Metab 2015;100(11):4133–9.
3. Avatapalle HB, Banerjee I, Shah S, et al. Abnormal neurodevelopmental outcomes are common in children with transient congenital hyperinsulinism. Front Endocrinol 2013;4:60.
4. James C, Kapoor RR, Ismail D, et al. The genetic basis of congenital hyperinsulinism. J Med Genet 2009;46(5):289–99.
5. Kalish JM, Boodhansingh KE, Bhatti TR, et al. Congenital hyperinsulinism in children with paternal 11p uniparental isodisomy and Beckwith-Wiedemann syndrome. J Med Genet 2016;53(1):53–61.
6. Hoe FM, Thornton PS, Wanner LA, et al. Clinical features and insulin regulation in infants with a syndrome of prolonged neonatal hyperinsulinism. J Pediatr 2006; 148(2):207–12.
7. Stanley CA, Rozance PJ, Thornton PS, et al. Re-evaluating "transitional neonatal hypoglycemia": mechanism and implications for management. J Pediatr 2015; 166(6):1520–5.e1.
8. Harris DL, Weston PJ, Harding JE. Incidence of neonatal hypoglycemia in babies identified as at risk. J Pediatr 2012;161(5):787–91.

9. McKinlay CJD, Alsweiler JM, Anstice NS, et al. Association of neonatal glycemia with neurodevelopmental outcomes at 4.5 years. JAMA Pediatr 2017;171(10): 972–83.

10. Thomas PM, Cote GJ, Wohllk N, et al. Mutations in the sulfonylurea receptor gene in familial persistent hyperinsulinemic hypoglycemia of infancy. Science 1995; 268(5209):426–9.

11. Thomas P, Ye Y, Lightner E. Mutation of the pancreatic islet inward rectifier Kir6.2 also leads to familial persistent hyperinsulinemic hypoglycemia of infancy. Hum Mol Genet 1996;5(11):1809–12.

12. De Leon D, Stanley CA. Pathophysiology of diffuse ATP-sensitive potassium channel hyperinsulinism. In: De Leon D, Stanley CA, editors. Monogenic hyperinsulinemic hypoglycemia disorders, vol. 21, 1st edition. Basel (Switzerland): Karger; 2012. p. 18–29.

13. Pinney SE, MacMullen C, Becker S, et al. Clinical characteristics and biochemical mechanisms of congenital hyperinsulinism associated with dominant KATP channel mutations. J Clin Invest 2008;118(8):2877–86.

14. Rahier J, Falt K, Muntefering H, et al. The basic structural lesion of persistent neonatal hypoglycaemia with hyperinsulinism: deficiency of pancreatic D cells or hyperactivity of B cells? Diabetologia 1984;26(4):282–9.

15. De Lonlay P, Fournet JC, Rahier J, et al. Somatic deletion of the imprinted 11p15 region in sporadic persistent hyperinsulinemic hypoglycemia of infancy is specific of focal adenomatous hyperplasia and endorses partial pancreatectomy. J Clin Invest 1997;100(4):802–7.

16. Verkarre V, Fournet JC, De Lonlay P, et al. Paternal mutation of the sulfonylurea receptor (SUR1) gene and maternal loss of 11p15 imprinted genes lead to persistent hyperinsulinism in focal adenomatous hyperplasia. J Clin Invest 1998;102(7): 1286–91.

17. Lord K, Dzata E, Snider KE, et al. Clinical presentation and management of children with diffuse and focal hyperinsulinism: a review of 223 cases. J Clin Endocrinol Metab 2013;98(11):E1786–9.

18. Snider KE, Becker S, Boyajian L, et al. Genotype and phenotype correlations in 417 children with congenital hyperinsulinism. J Clin Endocrinol Metab 2013; 98(2):E355–63.

19. Stanley CA, Lieu YK, Hsu BY, et al. Hyperinsulinism and hyperammonemia in infants with regulatory mutations of the glutamate dehydrogenase gene. N Engl J Med 1998;338(19):1352–7.

20. Bahi-Buisson N, Roze E, Dionisi C, et al. Neurological aspects of hyperinsulinism-hyperammonaemia syndrome. Dev Med Child Neurol 2008;50(12):945–9.

21. Glaser B, Kesavan P, Heyman M, et al. Familial hyperinsulinism caused by an activating glucokinase mutation. N Engl J Med 1998;338(4):226–30.

22. Sayed S, Langdon DR, Odili S, et al. Extremes of clinical and enzymatic phenotypes in children with hyperinsulinism caused by glucokinase activating mutations. Diabetes 2009;58(6):1419–27.

23. Pearson ER, Boj SF, Steele AM, et al. Macrosomia and hyperinsulinaemic hypoglycaemia in patients with heterozygous mutations in the HNF4A gene. PLoS Med 2007;4(4):e118.

24. Kapoor RR, Locke J, Colclough K, et al. Persistent hyperinsulinemic hypoglycemia and maturity-onset diabetes of the young due to heterozygous HNF4A mutations. Diabetes 2008;57(6):1659–63.

25. Stanescu DE, Hughes N, Kaplan B, et al. Novel presentations of congenital hyperinsulinism due to mutations in the MODY genes: HNF1A and HNF4A. J Clin Endocrinol Metab 2012;97(10):E2026–30.
26. Thornton PS, Stanley CA, De Leon DD, et al. Recommendations from the pediatric endocrine society for evaluation and management of persistent hypoglycemia in neonates, infants, and children. J Pediatr 2015;167(2):238–45.
27. Finegold DN, Stanley CA, Baker L. Glycemic response to glucagon during fasting hypoglycemia: an aid in the diagnosis of hyperinsulinism. J Pediatr 1980;96(2): 257–9.
28. Kelly A, Tang R, Becker S, et al. Poor specificity of low growth hormone and cortisol levels during fasting hypoglycemia for the diagnoses of growth hormone deficiency and adrenal insufficiency. Pediatrics 2008;122(3):e522–8.
29. Drash A, Wolff F. Drug therapy in leucine-sensitive hypoglycemia. Metab Clin Exp 1964;13:487–92.
30. Dayton PG, Pruitt AW, Faraj BA, et al. Metabolism and disposition of diazoxide. A mini-review. Drug Metab Dispos 1975;3(3):226–9.
31. Hirsch HJ, Loo S, Evans N, et al. Hypoglycemia of infancy and nesidioblastosis. Studies with somatostatin. N Engl J Med 1977;296(23):1323–6.
32. Laje P, Halaby L, Adzick NS, et al. Necrotizing enterocolitis in neonates receiving octreotide for the management of congenital hyperinsulinism. Pediatr Diabetes 2010;11(2):142–7.
33. Hawkes CP, Adzick NS, Palladino AA, et al. Late presentation of fulminant necrotizing enterocolitis in a child with hyperinsulinism on octreotide therapy. Horm Res Paediatr 2016;86(2):131–6.
34. Modan-Moses D, Koren I, Mazor-Aronovitch K, et al. Treatment of congenital hyperinsulinism with lanreotide acetate (Somatuline Autogel). J Clin Endocrinol Metab 2011;96(8):2312–7.
35. Kuhnen P, Marquard J, Ernert A, et al. Long-term lanreotide treatment in six patients with congenital hyperinsulinism. Horm Res Paediatr 2012;78(2):106–12.
36. Guemes M, Shah P, Silvera S, et al. Assessment of nifedipine therapy in hyperinsulinemic hypoglycemia due to mutations in the ABCC8 gene. J Clin Endocrinol Metab 2017;102(3):822–30.
37. Senniappan S, Alexandrescu S, Tatevian N, et al. Sirolimus therapy in infants with severe hyperinsulinemic hypoglycemia. N Engl J Med 2014;370(12):1131–7.
38. Szymanowski M, Estebanez MS, Padidela R, et al. mTOR inhibitors for the treatment of severe congenital hyperinsulinism: perspectives on limited therapeutic success. J Clin Endocrinol Metab 2016;101(12):4719–29.
39. Banerjee I, De Leon D, Dunne MJ. Extreme caution on the use of sirolimus for the congenital hyperinsulinism in infancy patient. Orphanet J Rare Dis 2017;12(1):70.
40. Stanley CA, Thornton PS, Ganguly A, et al. Preoperative evaluation of infants with focal or diffuse congenital hyperinsulinism by intravenous acute insulin response tests and selective pancreatic arterial calcium stimulation. J Clin Endocrinol Metab 2004;89(1):288–96.
41. Hardy OT, Hernandez-Pampaloni M, Saffer JR, et al. Accuracy of [18F]Fluorodopa positron emission tomography for diagnosing and localizing focal congenital hyperinsulinism. J Clin Endocrinol Metab 2007;92(12):4706–11.
42. Otonkoski T, Nanto-Salonen K, Seppanen M, et al. Noninvasive diagnosis of focal hyperinsulinism of infancy with [18F]-DOPA positron emission tomography. Diabetes 2006;55(1):13–8.
43. Laje P, States LJ, Zhuang H, et al. Accuracy of PET/CT Scan in the diagnosis of the focal form of congenital hyperinsulinism. J Pediatr Surg 2013;48(2):388–93.

44. Adzick NS, Thornton PS, Stanley CA, et al. A multidisciplinary approach to the focal form of congenital hyperinsulinism leads to successful treatment by partial pancreatectomy. J Pediatr Surg 2004;39(3):270–5.
45. Beltrand J, Caquard M, Arnoux JB, et al. Glucose metabolism in 105 children and adolescents after pancreatectomy for congenital hyperinsulinism. Diabetes Care 2012;35(2):198–203.
46. Menni F, de Lonlay P, Sevin C, et al. Neurologic outcomes of 90 neonates and infants with persistent hyperinsulinemic hypoglycemia. Pediatrics 2001;107(3): 476–9.

Congenital Hypopituitarism

John S. Parks, MD, PhD

KEYWORDS

- Hypopituitarism • Hypoglycemia • Cholestasis • Growth hormone • MRI
- Pituitary stalk • Guidelines

KEY POINTS

- Congenital hypopituitarism can be life threatening in neonates.
- A combination of prenatal, perinatal, and postnatal findings suggest the diagnosis. These findings include family history, brain or eye abnormalities, breech presentation, micropenis, hypoglycemia, and cholestasis.
- Most neonates with severe combined pituitary hormone deficiency show an ectopic posterior pituitary, abnormal pituitary stalk, and/or anterior pituitary hypoplasia on MRI.
- Characteristic MRI and low growth hormone (GH) levels in infancy establishes a diagnosis of GH deficiency. Recognition of adrenocorticotrophic hormone and/or thyroid-stimulating hormone deficiency establishes a diagnosis of combined pituitary hormone treatment and guides hormone replacement.

INTRODUCTION

Timely recognition of severe, congenital hypopituitarism is challenging. Short stature does not force consideration of the diagnosis, because birth weight and length are typically normal.[1–3] Clinicians must weigh a combination of family history, complications of pregnancy and delivery, physical findings, and postnatal problems such as hypoglycemia and jaundice in deciding whether to pursue the diagnosis. Once suspicion has been aroused, the pathway to diagnosis is fairly clear. It requires neuroimaging and selection of hormone assays to establish deficiency of growth hormone (GH) with or without insufficiency of other pituitary hormones. Early treatment can mitigate the metabolic and developmental consequences of hormone deficiencies, as well as providing the best chance of the infant's achieving a normal adult height.

CRUCIAL QUESTIONS ABOUT HYPOPITUITARISM

There are 3 crucial questions to ask when considering the possibility of congenital hypopituitarism.

Disclosure: The author has no commercial or financial conflicts of interest.
Emory University School of Medicine, Atlanta, GA 30322, USA
E-mail address: jsparks4410@gmail.com

Clin Perinatol 45 (2018) 75–91
https://doi.org/10.1016/j.clp.2017.11.001
0095-5108/18/© 2017 Elsevier Inc. All rights reserved.

What Hormones Are Missing?

Hypopituitarism involves underproduction of 1 or more of the 6 peptide hormones normally produced by 5 cell types in the anterior pituitary. There may be isolated deficiency of pituitary GH (IGHD) or combined pituitary hormone deficiency (CPHD) with additional deficiencies of thyroid-stimulating hormone (TSH), adrenocorticotrophic hormone (ACTH), prolactin (PRL), and the gonadotropins luteinizing hormone (LH) and follicle-stimulating hormone (FSH). There are also well-defined genetic disorders causing isolated deficiency of TSH,[4] ACTH,[5] and gonadotropins.[6] This article focuses on IGHD and CPHD.

Does MRI Show an Ectopic Posterior Pituitary?

MRI, introduced in the 1980s, provides detailed visualization of the anterior pituitary, the pituitary stalk, and the posterior pituitary bright spot.[7] Many children with congenital hypopituitarism show 1 or more of a triad of findings consisting of an ectopic posterior pituitary (EPP), anterior pituitary hypoplasia, and absence or attenuation of the stalk connecting the hypothalamus and pituitary. This combination is known as pituitary stalk interruption syndrome (PSIS).[8] It is a very common feature of CPHD. The triad is uncommon in IGHD, which is more commonly associated with isolated anterior pituitary hypoplasia or with normal MRI findings. PSIS identifies a subset of patients with IGHD who have a high risk for progression from IGHD to CPHD.[9]

Do Structural Abnormalities Extend Beyond the Pituitary Axis?

The most familiar association of abnormal hypothalamopituitary development with other central nervous system abnormalities is septo-optic dysplasia.[10] In this condition, hypopituitarism is linked to optic nerve hypoplasia and underdevelopment of the septum pellucidum. Other examples include anophthalmia, holoprosencephaly,[11] and Pallister-Hall syndrome,[12] an autosomal dominant disorder in which hypopituitarism is accompanied by hypothalamic hamartoma, polydactyly, imperforate anus, and renal anomalies. There is a risk of overlooking the component of hypopituitarism in infants with these complex conditions.

CATEGORIES OF HYPOPITUITARISM
Genetic Forms of Isolated Growth Hormone Deficiency

Congenital isolated GH deficiency (GHD) has an incidence of 1 in 4000 to 1 in 10,000 live births. There are several well-characterized genetic forms that show autosomal recessive, autosomal dominant, or X-linked patterns of inheritance and these are termed type 1-A, type 1-B, type 2, and type 3 (**Table 1**).[13] Type 1-A shows complete absence of GH and is caused by deletions or complete loss-of-function mutations of the GH1 gene.[14] It was initially recognized in Swiss children with extremely short stature who developed antibodies that neutralized GH effects when treated with extracted pituitary GH.[15] Subsequent reports indicated that anti-GH antibody formation is a variable feature of this condition.[16] Type 1-B refers to a less severe phenotype. One form is caused by missense mutations or by splice site mutations that eliminate the fourth exon of the GH1 gene.[17] A similar phenotype is produced by mutations in the GHRHR gene encoding the pituitary receptor for the hypothalamic GH-releasing hormone.[18] Type 2 is a dominant form of IGHD. Mutations of the GH1 gene account for more than 80% of dominant IGHD. Most common are splice donor site mutations that exclude

Table 1
Causes of neonatal hypopituitarism

	Heredity	Comments
IGHD		
GH1 gene deletions or mutations 1-A	AR	Severe, ±anti-GH antibodies
GH1 gene mutations 1-B	AR	Less severe
GHRHR gene mutations 1-B	AR	Less severe
GH1 gene mutations 2	AD	Maternal and fetal IGHD
BTK 3	XL	Very rare
CPHD		
PROP1 mutations GH, TSH, PRL, ACTH, LH, FSH	AR	Common in eastern Europe
POU1F1 mutations GH, TSH, PRL	AR	First transcription factor disease
POU1F1 (R271W) GH, TSH, PRL	AD	Risk of maternal/fetal hypothyroidism
LHX3 mutations GH, TSH, PRL, ACTH	AR	Rigid cervical spine
LHX4 mutations GH, TSH, ACTH, LH, FSH	AD	Small sella, ±EPP, Chiari malformation
IGHD or CPHD with PSIS		
Pituitary stalk interruption syndrome	Complex	IGHD may progress to CPHD
Pituitary aplasia	Complex	Severe CPHD, early expression
Syndromic conditions that include PSIS		
Septo-optic dysplasia	Complex	Variable midbrain abnormalities
Holoprosencephaly	Complex	Also at risk for diabetes insipidus
Microphthalmia/anophthalmia OTX2, *SOX2*	Complex	CPHD in 1 in 3
Pallister-Hall syndrome *GLI3*	AD	Hypothalamic hamartoma, bifid epiglottis

Abbreviations: ACTH, adrenocorticotrophic hormone; AD, autosomal dominant; AR, autosomal recessive; CPHD, combined pituitary hormone deficiency; EPP, ectopic posterior pituitary; FSH, follicle-stimulating hormone; GH, growth hormone; LH, luteinizing hormone; IGHD, isolated growth hormone deficiency; PSIS, pituitary stalk interruption syndrome; TSH, thyroid-stimulating hormone; XL, X linked.

exon 3 from messenger RNA and eliminate amino acids 32 to 71 of the 191 amino acid protein.[19] The mutant protein interferes with expression of the normal allele.[20] X-linked recessive IGHD3 is less well understood. Most cases have been associated with immunoglobulin deficiency and linked to the Bruton thymidine kinase *BTK* gene on chromosome Xq27.1.[21] MRI shows a normal to small anterior pituitary gland, eutopic posterior pituitary, and normal stalk in these simple genetic forms of IGHD.[22]

Genetic Forms of Combined Pituitary Hormone Deficiency Without Pituitary Stalk Interruption Syndrome

These nonsyndromic genetic forms of CPHD involve mutations of genes that direct the cascade of events leading to the emergence and continued function of hormone-producing anterior pituitary cells. Two genes, *PROP1* and *POU1F1* (also known as *PIT1* and *GHF1*), are particularly important in this regard. *PROP1* expression precedes and is necessary for the later expression of *Pit-1*, earning it the name prophet of Pit-1. Mutation results in CPHD involving GH, TSH, PRL, ACTH, LH, and FSH.[23] The evolution of hormone deficiencies is typically delayed and progressive with clinical recognition of GHD around age 5 years, preceding recognition of TSH and gonadotropin deficiency.[24] In Bottner and colleagues'[25] series of 9 patients with a mean follow-up interval of 15 years, GH replacement was begun at age 6.1 years, thyroid hormone at 6.8 years, sex hormones at 15.0 years, and all required hydrocortisone replacement, at a mean age of 18.4 years. There is, however, considerable variation in timing and severity of hormone deficiencies, even among affected siblings with homozygosity for the same mutation. Some affected individuals have presented with central hypothyroidism within the first month of life.[26] The anterior pituitary gland may be small as expected in CPHD, normal, large, or very large.[27,28] It is common to develop an intrapituitary mass that is initially solid, becomes cystic, and regresses over time without surgical intervention.[24]

Mutations of the POU1F1 gene cause deficiencies of GH, TSH, and PRL.[29] ACTH and gonadotropin production are normal. The GHD is severe. Untreated, it typically leads to severe short stature within the first year. The severity of TSH deficiency is variable, ranging from severe congenital hypothyroidism[29] to mild central hypothyroidism identified in midchildhood.[30] The anterior pituitary is small or of normal size.[30]

PROP1 mutations are a much more common cause of CPHD than are POU1F1 mutations, by a factor more than 10:1 in most series. In 2015, De Rienzo and colleagues[31] reported the frequencies of genetic defects in Italian patients with CPHD and in similar surveys from other countries. PROP1 mutations accounted for 6.7% of sporadic cases and 48.5% of families with 2 or more affected children. POU1F1 mutations accounted for 1.6% of sporadic and 21.6% of familial cases. The frequencies of HESX1, LHX3, and LHX4 mutations were each less than 1%.

Although there are many types of PROP1 mutations, 2 are much more common than the others. They are c.301-302delAG and c150delA, which each cause a shift in reading frame and preclude synthesis of functional Prop1 protein. Originally thought to be hot spots for recurrent mutation, the high rates of these mutations in Polish, Russian, Lithuanian, and Hungarian CPHD, and rarity in patients from western European and Asia, suggested a founder effect.[32,33] Haplotype analysis in 231 patients from 21 countries indicated that the 2-base-pair deletion originated in the region of Lithuania about 2500 years ago.[33] The haplotype diverged in the region of the Iberian peninsula about 500 years ago and spread to Brazil. The 1-base-pair deletion had its ancestral origin in the region of Belarus about 1100 years ago.

All of the PROP1 mutations are recessive. Most of the POU1F1 mutations are also recessive, but there is also a fairly common dominant mutation. It involves substitution of tryptophan for arginine at position 171. The combination of an affected mother and an affected fetus sets the stage for severe intrauterine hypothyroidism to occur if the mother does not receive appropriate thyroid hormone replacement during pregnancy. Two particularly instructive cases were reported 18 years apart.[34,35] In one, the mother was noncompliant in taking her levothyroxine. In the other, the obstetrician interpreted a low TSH value in the second trimester as a sign of overtreatment and reduced levothyroxine to about one-third of what is needed in pregnancy. Both term newborns had much more severe intrauterine hypothyroidism than the usual primary congenital hypothyroidism. They experienced severe respiratory distress and were developmentally delayed.

Combined Pituitary Hormone Deficiency or Isolated Deficiency of Pituitary Growth Hormone with Pituitary Stalk Interruption Syndrome

As mentioned earlier, the PSIS represents the MRI findings of an EPP bright spot together with a small or absent pituitary stalk and a hypoplastic anterior pituitary gland. In sagittal views, with T1-weighted imaging, the neurohypophysis is normally seen as a bright spot. This brightness is thought to be caused by storage of vasopressin–neurophysin II copeptin complexes made in hypothalamic neurons and transported by long axons through the stalk to the posterior pituitary. An EPP can reside in the hypothalamus or at any point along the pituitary stalk.

The stalk is surrounded by a portal venous network connecting a venous plexus in the hypothalamus to another venous plexus in the anterior pituitary. Interruption of the vascular supply deprives the anterior pituitary cells of releasing and release-inhibiting hormones, resulting in a hypoplastic and hypofunctioning gland.

Regulation of vasopressin release from the truncated stalk is generally normal, in contrast with tumor encroachment or surgical transection of the stalk, which produces retrograde degeneration of hypothalamic neurons and causes diabetes insipidus.

Several important conclusions can be drawn from the many clinical studies of PSIS (**Box 1**). Triulzi and colleagues[36] examined 101 pediatric patients with hypopituitarism and found that 59% had EPP. Among those with EPP, 49% had CPHD. Among those without EPP, 12% had CPHD.

The proportion of CPHD is even higher when focusing on children diagnosed at an early age. In a 2015 article entitled "Brain Magnetic Resonance Imaging as a First-line Investigation for Growth Hormone Deficiency Diagnosis in Early Childhood," Pampanini and colleagues[37] focused on a series of 68 children with hypopituitarism who presented at 2 pediatric hospitals in Rome before 4 years of age. All of the 31 with CPHD had EPP. Of the 37 with IGHD, 35% had EPP, 49% had isolated pituitary hypoplasia, and only 16% had normal MRI studies. Most of the children with IGHD and normal pituitary anatomy were more than 24 months old at time of diagnosis. Hamilton and colleagues[38] assessed the relationship between PSIS and the severity of GHD. Among patients with IGHD with severe GHD, defined as peak stimulated GH levels less than 3 μg/L, the frequency of PSIS was 90%. Among those with peaks of 3 to 9 μg/L, the frequency of PSIS was 39%. Tauber and colleagues[39] reported on follow-up and treatment of children with PSIS. They observed conversion from IGHD to CPHD in their patients, such that those who had reached maturity all had GHD and 2 or 3 other anterior pituitary hormone deficiencies. From a more global perspective, more than 5% of 1757 children who were originally diagnosed with idiopathic IGHD and followed in the Lilly GeNeSIS observational study for more than

---

Box 1
Principles of pituitary stalk interruption syndrome

- PSIS accounts for most cases of congenital CPHD
- PSIS is also seen in children with severe IGHD
- Children with severe IGHD and PSIS are at risk for developing CPHD
- PSIS is a feature of several other conditions, including septo-optic dysplasia
- The genetic contributions to PSIS are complex

4 years developed 1 or more additional deficiencies.[40] As in the follow-up of children with PROP1 mutations, surveillance for life-threatening ACTH deficiency needs to be maintained.

Syndromic Conditions That Include Pituitary Stalk Interruption Syndrome

A recent review of the genetics of CPHD suggests that CPHD is a spectrum disorder, with holoprosencephaly and septo-optic dysplasia (SOD) at the severe end, CPHD with PSIS in the middle, and IGHD and hypogonadotropic hypogonadism at the mild end.[41] The eye, ear, nose, anterior pituitary gland, and some cranial nerve ganglia share common developmental programs. Disruption is probably multifactorial, with environmental as well as genetic influences. It may also be bigenic or oligogenic, with heterozygosity for mutations in 2 or more genes being responsible for disease. The discovery of homozygosity for a HESX1 mutation in siblings with SOD opened a fresh window on a genetic cause but turned out to be an uncommon explanation for the condition.[42] The number of candidate genes associated with hypopituitarism increased by 1 or 2 per year from the discovery of POU1F1 in 1992 through recognition of FGF8 mutations in CPHD and Kallmann syndrome in 2011.[41] There are now more than 30 genes to consider, with the rate of discovery accelerating through application of whole exome sequencing. OTX2 and SOX2 mutations have produced microphthalmia/anophthalmia and CPHD. GLI3 mutations can cause Pallister-Hall syndrome. Several genes in the sonic hedgehog pathway contribute to nonsyndromic PSIS, as they do to holoprosencephaly.[43] As of mid-2017, more than 80% of instances of CPHD, with or without PSIS and extrapituitary abnormalities, have not been explained at the genetic level.

Prenatal and Perinatal Infections

Anterior as well as posterior pituitary failure needs to be considered in the setting of overwhelming sepsis. An increase of serum sodium level together with an inappropriately high urine output establishes the diagnosis of diabetes insipidus. Deficiencies of ACTH, TSH, and GH may develop acutely or long after recovery from the infection. This course of events has been described for group B streptococcal salmonella infections.[44,45] Battered neonates are also at risk for diabetes insipidus accompanied by anterior hypopituitarism.[46]

REASONS TO SUSPECT HYPOPITUITARISM

Suspicion of congenital GHD or CPHD can be aroused by many things. Some of the more important features are outlined in **Box 2**.

A family history of hypopituitarism suggests that the fetus is at increased risk. Normal parents and an affected sibling suggest the possibility of a recessive or polygenic disorder. An affected parent may have passed on a dominant disorder such as IGHD3 or a dominant mutation in the POU1F1 gene. An affected maternal uncle raises the issue of X-linked inheritance. It is important to obtain detailed pedigree and phenotype information to understand the potential risks to mother and fetus.

Breech presentation has a long history of association with hypothyroidism. In 1977, Rona and Tanner[47] summarized their experience in England and Wales as well as earlier studies in the United States, France, and Switzerland. The frequency of breech delivery was 8.9% in 168 cases of IGHD and 42.3% in 85 cases of CPHD, compared with a frequency of 2.5% in first-born and 1.9% in later-born infants in the general population. There was no doubt about an

---

Box 2
Reasons to suspect hypopituitarism

Prenatal

- Positive family history. Particularly mother, also siblings and cousins.
- Breech presentation. A result rather than a cause of PSIS.
- Midline brain abnormalities on ultrasonography. Septo-optic dysplasia and others.
- Not fetal growth retardation.

Prenatal by ultrasonography or postnatal by physical examination

- Cleft palate, single central incisor. Consider holoprosencephaly.
- Micropenis less than 2 cm, undescended testes in boys. GHD or CPHD.

Postnatal

- Low T4 level with normal TSH level on newborn screen.
- Hypoglycemia plus or minus seizures. Severe, early, and sustained.
- Jaundice. Initially unconjugated. Cholestasis within weeks if ACTH deficient.
- Optic nerve hypoplasia. Nystagmus evident by 3 months.
- Growth failure. Length typically −3 standard deviations by age 12 months.

---

association, but the investigators stated succinctly that "The problem is to know whether the fetus was normal before delivery started."[47] They argued that micropenis in boys was an indication of a process that began well before birth. Others documented a high frequency of breech deliveries and forceps deliveries in children with idiopathic CPHD and argued that perinatal trauma caused hypothalamic damage.[48] The association has persisted into an era of MRI for PSIS and routine cesarean section for breech presentation. There is general acceptance that something about the fetus is predisposing to this complication, in common with fetuses with Prader-Willi, who have a similar incidence of breech presentation.[49]

Midline brain abnormalities, including absence of the septum pellucidum and absence of the corpus callosum, may foretell septo-optic dysplasia. Cleft palate or a single central incisor may be identified prenatally, prompting consideration of hypopituitarism associated with holoprosencephaly. Micropenis, without hypospadias and with a length of less than 2 cm at term, is seen in both IGHD and CPHD.

The combination of low total T4 and inappropriately low TSH level is identified in state programs that test for both T4 and TSH in screening protocols for primary congenital hypothyroidism.

Neonatal hypoglycemia is seen in both GHD and CPHD but tends to be more severe when there is ACTH deficiency. Symptoms include lethargy and seizures. The clinical picture resembles hyperinsulinemic hypoglycemia with early onset, persistence beyond 3 days of age, requirement for high glucose infusion rates to maintain normoglycemia, and inability to tolerate a normal interval between feedings. Insulin levels are helpful in excluding hyperinsulinism and focusing on hypopituitarism.

Binder and colleagues[50] described the course of neonatal cholestasis in 9 infants with CPHD diagnosed in a single institution over an interval of

25 years. The condition was recognized at a median age of 13 days and resolved with hormone replacement at a median age of 88 days. Maximum direct bilirubin level averaged 6.9 mg/dL with a range of 2.4 to 11.6 mg/dL. Alkaline phosphatase level was high, transaminase levels were minimally increased, and gamma glutamyl transferase level was generally normal. Liver biopsies, done in 4 infants before the diagnosis of CPHD, showed canalicular cholestasis and mild portal eosinophilic infiltration but not portal fibrosis. All of the children had central hypothyroidism and cortisol deficiency, with mean cortisol levels of 1.5 μg/dL at the time of hypoglycemia. All had elements of PSIS on MRI. None developed chronic liver disease. The combination of hypoglycemia and cholestasis should definitely prompt suspicion of CPHD or isolated ACTH deficiency.[51]

CASE PRESENTATION

Fig. 1 shows sagittal and coronal MRI of a 12-day-old boy with congenital hypopituitarism. The MRI shows an EPP, attenuated pituitary stalk, and a normal anterior pituitary gland with a height of 3 mm. Other images show small optic nerves and optic chiasm. The corpus callosum and septum pellucidum were normal. There was absence of the right olfactory nerve.

The patient was born at gestational age 39 weeks by elective cesarean section because of a maternal history of repeated miscarriages associated with hypercoaglability. Birth weight and length were normal. Features leading to suspicion of hypopituitarism included micropenis, blood glucose of 30 mg/dL on day 1 responding to hydrocortisone replacement, and an abnormally low total T4 level with normal TSH level on newborn metabolic screening. The total T4 level on day 2 was 6 μg/dL. At 7 days of age, total T4 was 2.9 μg/dL; free T4, 0.8 ng/mL; and TSH, 6.0 mIU/L. He was admitted to a pediatric hospital at age 11 days because of poor feeding, weight loss, lethargy, and jaundice. On admission, serum electrolyte levels were normal. Total bilirubin level was 13.9 mg/dL and direct bilirubin was 0.2 mg/dL. Aspartate transaminase and alanine transaminase levels were increased. Low-dose (1 μg) ACTH stimulation showed a peak cortisol level of 7.1 μg/dL. Serum GH level was 3.37 μg/L at 14 days of age.

This brief summary of a newborn infant with optic nerve hypoplasia and hypopituitarism shows the importance of clinical signs and symptoms suggesting a diagnosis. Criteria for refining the diagnosis and beginning treatment are addressed later.

GUIDELINES FOR DIAGNOSIS OF CONGENITAL GROWTH HORMONE DEFICIENCY AND COMBINED PITUITARY HORMONE DEFICIENCY

In 2016, Grimberg and colleagues[52] published a new set of guidelines for GH and insulinlike growth factor I (IGF-I) treatment of children and adolescents. The recommendations were a joint effort of the Drug and Therapeutics Committee and the Ethics Committee of the Pediatric Endocrine Society. Section 2.1.2 is particularly relevant: "We suggest that GHD due to congenital hypopituitarism be diagnosed without formal GH provocative testing in a newborn with hypoglycemia who does not attain a serum GH concentration above 5 μg/L and who has deficiency of at least one additional pituitary hormone and/or the classical imaging triad (ectopic posterior pituitary and pituitary hypoplasia with abnormal stalk).[52] The guidelines also state as a technical remark that "A low GH

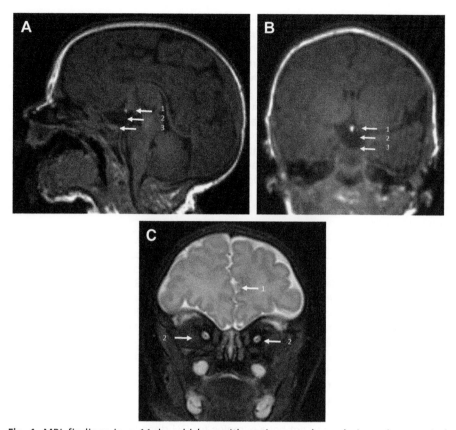

Fig. 1. MRI findings in a 14-day-old boy with optic nerve hypoplasia and congenital hypopituitarism. (*A*) Sagittal T1 weighted image. (*Arrow 1*) T1 hyperintense focus represents the EPP bright spot, abnormally located at the floor of the third ventricle. (*Arrow 2*) Attenuated pituitary stalk. (*Arrow 3*) Anterior pituitary gland. (*B*) Coronal T1 weighted image. (*Arrow 1*) EPP bright spot. (*Arrow 2*) Decreased visualization of pituitary stalk. (*Arrow 3*) Anterior pituitary gland. Incidentally, the cavum septum pellucidum is present in this neonate. (*C*) Coronal T2 weighted image. (*Arrow 1*) Absence of anterior falx, allowing interdigitation of frontal gyri. (*Arrows 2*) Symmetrically small optic nerves. Also noted on image, absence of the right olfactory nerve. (*Courtesy of* Sarah Milla, MD, Children's Healthcare of Atlanta, Atlanta, GA.)

concentration at the time of hypoglycemia is alone insufficient to diagnose GHD."[52]

DIAGNOSTIC TESTS
Neuroimaging

MRI is the preferred modality for assessing the hypothalamic and pituitary region in infants and young children.[53] Recommended protocols involve 2-mm to 3-mm thick, high-resolution T1-weighted and T2-weighted images in both the coronal and the sagittal planes. Anterior pituitary size and contour as well as the size and location of the posterior pituitary bright spot are well visualized in sagittal T1 images. Coronal images are excellent for seeing the anterior pituitary, stalk, chiasm, and parasellar regions. Dynamic imaging with contrast provides further information about the vascular component of the pituitary stalk.[54] Axial T2-weighted imaging of the whole brain is recommended to look for other abnormalities. A typical evaluation includes qualitative description and height measurement for the anterior pituitary; location and dimensions of the posterior pituitary bright spot; description of the pituitary stalk, optic chiasm, septum pellucidum, and corpus callosum; and statements about abnormality of other brain structures. There are important concerns about practicality and safety of MRI imaging in tertiary as well as primary hospital settings. Tocchio and colleagues[55] published a detailed update on "MRI Evaluation and Safety in the Developing Brain" in the April 2015 issue of *Seminars in Perinatology*. Although not specifically addressing pituitary imaging, it addresses important issues of 3-T vs 1.5-T field strength, transportation and monitoring of neonates, and sedation, and of special equipment for neonatal imaging.

Growth Hormone

The diagnosis of GHD in older children usually requires subnormal GH values in all samples obtained during 2 or more GH stimulation tests. Such tests, using insulin, glucagon, levodopa, clonidine, arginine, or other agents, are considered dangerous and are contraindicated in newborns and young infants. Alternatives to stimulation tests involve assay of random specimens obtained during the first week and specimens obtained at the time of hypoglycemia.

Serum GH hormone levels are high in normal term infants during the first week after birth.[56] Leger and colleagues[57] observed a mean GH level of 29 ± 17 µg/L in 36 infants at 3 days of age and Vavarigou and colleagues[58] reported similar findings with a mean of 24 ± 12.3 µg/L in 30 infants at 3 days of age. The numbers of subjects are low and the standard deviations are broad. Furthermore, many infants with suspected GHD may not have samples for GH done in the first week. Binder and colleagues[59] addressed both issues by doing GH assays on eluates from dried blood spots on filter paper cards used for newborn metabolic screening. Geometric mean values on 269 samples obtained at 3 to 5 days were 15.4 µg/L for boys and 17.5 µg/L for girls. Retrospective analysis of stored newborn screening specimens from 9 patients with CPHD and malformation of the pituitary gland ranged from 0.8 to 5.5 µg/L, providing a cutoff value of 7 µg/L for the polyclonal GH enzyme-linked immunosorbent assay used in this study. A subsequent study, which adjusted for longer durations of storage for screening cards, confirmed subnormal GH values during the neonatal period in children with delayed diagnoses of CPHD but showed normal values in children with IGHD.[60] It seems that random sampling of GH in the first week is helpful in establishing a diagnosis of GHD whether done prospectively, retroactively on stored serum specimens obtained for other purposes, or on eluates from newborn screening cards.

GH and cortisol levels are frequently measured at the time of hypoglycemia. Although low values can be used to support a diagnosis of GHD or CPHD, they lack specificity. Kelly and colleagues[61] reviewed the Children's Hospital of Philadelphia experience with fasting studies done to investigate suspected hypoglycemia in 151 children. Some 84 children became hypoglycemic with blood glucose levels less than or equal to 50 mg/dL. GH values were less than a normal cutoff of 7.5 µg/L in 70% and cortisol values were less than a normal cutoff of 18 µg/L in 61% of critical specimens. The 1 GH-deficient child in the series had GH and cortisol levels just less than the cutoff limits. In an analysis of fasting studies in 31 infants with hyerinsulinemic hypoglycemia, Seniappan and Hussain[62] found that 35% had GH values less than 7.5 mg/L. The mean cortisol level was low at 7.3 μg/dL and the mean insulin level of 11.9 mU/L was at the end of the fast.

Adrenocorticotrophic Hormone and Cortisol

The diagnosis of complete ACTH deficiency is supported by baseline cortisol levels of less than 2.2 μg/dL and low ACTH levels. Partial ACTH deficiency is suggested by baseline cortisol of 2.2 to 8.0 μg/dL and low ACTH level. Early morning sampling is preferred after a diurnal pattern of cortisol levels is established around 2 months of age. Mehta and colleagues[63] compared standard Synacthen stimulation and sampling at 0 and 30 minutes with cortisol sampling every 2 hours for 24 hours in 28 children at risk for ACTH deficiency. Most of the children had a diagnosis of septo-optic dysplasia and half were less than a year of age when tested. The investigators concluded that the combination of an 08:00 serum cortisol level greater than 6.3 μg/dL and a 30-minute serum cortisol level greater than 20 μg/dL would ensure that no child with ACTH would be missed and experience serious consequences, but that these results could lead to overdiagnosis of ACTH deficiency. Maghnie and colleagues[64] compared insulin-induced hypoglycemia, low-dose ACTH, standard ACTH, and corticotropin-releasing hormone stimulation tests. A low morning cortisol level and a subnormal response to the physiologically low-dose Synacthen test emerged as the best indicators of an intact axis.

Thyroid Hormone

The diagnosis of central hypothyroidism is made by finding a low fT4 level with an inappropriately low TSH level. Studies from the 1990s often refer to the criterion of a low or delayed TSH response to thyrotropin-releasing hormone, which is no longer available for diagnostic use in the United States.

Sex Hormones

Normal male infants experience a surge in LH, FSH, and testosterone levels that is evident by 1 week and lasts for several 4 to 6 months after birth.[65] This surge provides a window of opportunity for evaluation of the hypothalamic-pituitary-gonadal axis. Braslavsky and colleagues[66] examined the association between micropenis and/or undescended testes and LH, FSH, testosterone, antimullerian hormone (AMH), and inhibin-B levels in 27 boys with hypoglycemia and/or cholestasis referred for evaluation of possible hypopituitarism. The ages at hormonal assessment ranged from 0.5 to 6 months. All but 1 of the 15 boys with CPHD and genital hypoplasia had abnormally low LH and testosterone levels compared with those with CPHD and normal genitalia, and with the small number without hypopituitarism. FSH, AMH, and inhibin-B levels were similar in the 3 groups. The investigators suggest that a combination of detailed evaluation of the external genital phenotype together with assessment of LH and testosterone levels during the postnatal surge of gonadotropins facilitates the diagnosis of hypogonadotropic hypogonadism at an early age. This information can help in deciding whether and when to start testosterone or LH-releasing hormone treatment.

Genetic Tests

DNA testing can be useful in diagnosis, genetic counseling, and providing continuing coverage for cases of suspected monogenic IGHD and CPHD. Athena Diagnostics, for example, provides a Short Stature panel that includes *GH1*, *GHRHR* (growth hormone releasing hormone receptor), and *SHOX* (short stature homeobox) sequencing. Their CPHD, Pituitary Disorder panel tests for mutations in *POU1F1* and *PROP1*. Components of these panels can be ordered individually. They are more helpful in familial than in sporadic hypopituitarism. The genetic contributions to PSIS are too complex to cover in a sequencing panel. It is hoped that, with networking among investigators for discovery and verification of the expanding number of genes associated with severe congenital hypopituitarism, more generally applicable panels will emerge.

MANAGEMENT

GH replacement involves daily subcutaneous injections of recombinant human GH at a dosage between 0.16 and 0.24 mg/kg/week. Glucocorticoid replacement should be begun before thyroid hormone replacement because of the risk that restoration of a euthyroid state can destabilize a patient with ACTH deficiency. Hydrocortisone dose should be given in a minimum of 3 doses a day for a total dose of 8 to 12 mg/m^2/d for maintenance, and 2 or 3 times that for stress/illness. Levothyroxine dose is similar to that used in congenital primary hypothyroidism. Reliance should be placed on achieving free T4 concentrations in the upper third of normal, rather than on TSH levels in deciding on dose adjustments. Infants with cholestasis may need higher doses of hydrocortisone and levothyroxine because of malabsorption.[67]

Management requires interdisciplinary teamwork from a spectrum of clinicians including perinatologists, neonatologists, pediatric endocrinologists, geneticists, and often neurologists and ophthalmologists. A useful adage is that multidisciplinary teams see the patients and their families, but interdisciplinary teams also understand and communicate with each other.

Best Practices

What is the condition?

Congenital hypopituitarism

What is the current practice?

Recognition is often delayed until growth failure develops in later childhood, despite telltale signs such as hypoglycemia and jaundice as neonates.

Diagnosis of GHD is made through stimulation tests, followed by MRI evaluation.

What changes in current practice are likely to improve outcomes?

Develop a suspicion of hypopituitarism based on prenatal, perinatal, and postnatal clues, especially hypoglycemia.

Assess GH, cortisol, and thyroid hormone levels in basal specimens.

Proceed to MRI evaluation looking for an EPP, abnormal pituitary stalk, and/or hypoplastic anterior pituitary.

A clinical algorithm is included as **Fig. 2**.

Rating of the strength of evidence is 2 out of 4 based on 2016 taskforce recommendations by Geysenbergh and colleagues.[49]

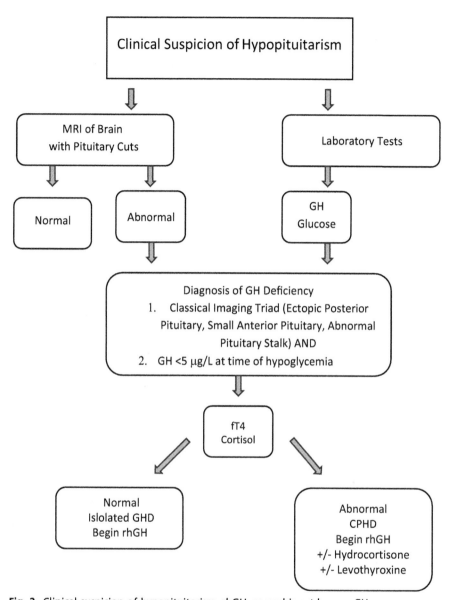

Fig. 2. Clinical suspicion of hypopituitarism. rhGH, recombinant human GH.

REFERENCES

1. Mullis P-E, Tonella P. Regulation of fetal growth: consequences and impact of being born small. Best Pract Res Clin Endocrinol Metab 2008;22:173–90.
2. Parks JS. The ontogeny of growth hormone sensitivity. Horm Res 2001;55(Suppl 2):27–31.
3. Netchine I, Assi S, Le Bouc Y, et al. IGF-I molecular anomalies demonstrate its critical role in fetal, postnatal growth and brain development. Best Pract Res Clin Endocrinol Metab 2011;25:181–90.

4. Schoenmakers N, Alatzoglou KS, Chatterjee VK, et al. Recent advances in central congenital hypothyroidism. J Endocrinol 2015;227:R51–71.

5. Couture C, Saveanu A, Barlier A, et al. Phenotypic homogeneity and genotypic variability in a large series of congenital isolated ACTH-deficiency patients with TPIT mutations. J Clin Endocrinol Metab 2012;97:E486–95.

6. Boehm U, Bouloux PM, Dattani M, et al. Expert consensus document: European consensus on congenital hypogonadotropic hypogonadism-pathogenesis, diagnosis and treatment. Nat Rev Endocrinol 2015;11:547–64.

7. Pressman BD. Pituitary imaging. Endocrinol Metab Clin N Am 2017;46:713–48.

8. Scotti G, Triulzi F, Chiumello G, et al. New imaging techniques in endocrinology: magnetic resonance of the pituitary gland and sella turcica. Acta Paediatr Scand 1989;365:5–14.

9. Maghnie M, Mengarda F, Sartirana P, et al. Long-term follow-up evaluation of magnetic resonance imaging in the prognosis of permanent GH deficiency. Eur J Endocrinol 2000;143:493–6.

10. Garcia-Filion P, Borchert M. Optic nerve hypoplasia syndrome: a review of the epidemiology and clinical associations. Curr Treat Options Neurol 2013;15: 78–89.

11. Kaliaperumal C, Ndoro S, Mandiwanza T, et al. Holoprosencephaly: antenatal and postnatal diagnosis and outcome. Childs Nerv Syst 2016;32:801–9.

12. Hall JG. Pallister-Hall syndrome has gone the way of modern medical genetics. Am J Med Genet C Semin Med Genet 2014;166C:414–8.

13. Di Lorgi N, Morana G, Allegri AEM, et al. Classical and non-classical causes of GH deficiency in the paediatric age. Best Pract Res Clin Endocrinol Metab 2016;30:705–36.

14. Phillips JA III, Hjelle BL, Seeburg PH, et al. Molecular basis for familial isolated growth hormone deficiency. Proc Natl Acad Sci U S A 1981;78:6372–5.

15. Illig R. Growth hormone antibodies in patients treated with different preparations of human growth hormone (HGH). Lancet 1970;6:679–88.

16. Laron Z, Kelijman M, Pertzelan A, et al. Human growth hormone gene deletion without antibody formation or growth arrest during treatment–a new disease entity? Isr J Med Sci 1985;21:999–1006.

17. Proctor AM, Phillips JA, Cooper DN. The molecular genetics of growth hormone deficiency. Hum Genet 1998;103:255–72.

18. Wajnrajch MP, Gertner JM, Harbison MD, et al. Nonsense mutation in the human growth hormone-releasing hormone receptor causes growth failure analogous to the little (lit) mouse. Nat Genet 1996;12:88–90.

19. Mosely CT, Mullis PE, Prince MA, et al. An exon splice enhancer mutation causes autosomal dominant GH deficiency. J Clin Endocrinol Metab 2002;87:847–52.

20. Mullis PE, Deladoey J, Dannies PS. Molecular and cellular basis of isolated dominant-negative growth hormone deficiency, IGHD type II: insights on the secretory pathway of peptide hormones. Horm Res 2002;58:53–66.

21. Stewart DM, Tian L, Notarangelo LD, et al. X-linked hypogammaglobulinemia and isolated growth hormone deficiency: an update. Immunol Res 2008;40:262–70.

22. Komreich L, Horev G, Lazar L, et al. MR findings in hereditary isolated growth hormone deficiency. Am J Neuroradiol 1997;18:1743–7.

23. Wu W, Cogan JD, Pfaffle RW, et al. Mutations in PROP1 cause familial combined pituitary hormone deficiency. Nat Genet 1998;18:147–9.

24. Mody S, Brown MR, Parks JS. The spectrum of hypopituitarism caused by Prop1 mutations. Best Pract Res Clin Endocrinol Metab 2002;16:421–31.

25. Bottner A, Keller E, Kratzsch J, et al. PROP1 mutations cause progressive deterioration of anterior pituitary function. J Clin Endocrinol Metab 2004;89:5256–65.

26. Voutetakis A, Maniati-Cristaldi M, Kanaka-Gantenbein C, et al. Prolonged jaundice and hypothyroidism as the presenting symptoms in a neonate with a novel Prop 1 gene mutation (Q83X). Eur J Endocrinol 2004;150:257–64.

27. Obermannova B, Pfaeffle R, Zygmunt-Gorskaa A, et al. Mutations and pituitary morphology in a series of patients with PROP1 gene defects. Horm Res Paediatr 2011;76:348–54.

28. Parks JS, Tenore A, Bongiovanni AM, et al. Familial hypopituitarism with large sella turcica. N Engl J Med 1977;298:698–702.

29. Tatsumi K, Kiyai K, Notomi T, et al. Cretinism with combined hormone deficiency caused by a mutation in the PIT1 gene. Nat Genet 1992;1:56–8.

30. Pfaffle RW, DiMattia G, Parks JS, et al. Mutation of the POU-specific domain of Pit-1 and hypopituitarism without pituitary hypoplasia. Science 1992;257:1118–21.

31. De Rienzo F, Mellone S, Bellone S, et al. Frequency of genetic defects in combined pituitary hormone deficiency: a systematic review and analysis of a multicenter Italian cohort. Clin Endocrinol 2015;83:849–60.

32. Deladoey J, Fluck C, Buyukgebiz A, et al. "Hot spot" in the PROP1 gene responsible for combined pituitary hormone deficiency. J Clin Endocrinol Metab 1999; 84:1645–50.

33. Dusatkova P, Pfaffle R, Brown MR, et al. Genesis of two most prevalent PROP1 gene variants causing combined pituitary hormone deficiency in 21 populations. Eur J Hum Genet 2016;24:415–20.

34. De Zegher F, Pernasetti F, Vanhole C, et al. The prenatal role of thyroid hormone evidenced by fetomaternal Pit-1 deficiency. J Clin Endocrinol Metab 1995;80: 3127–30.

35. Pine-Twaddell E, Romero CJ, Radovick S. Vertical transmission of hypopituitarism: critical importance of appropriate interpretation of thyroid function tests and levothyroxine therapy during pregnancy. Thyroid 2013;23:892–7.

36. Triulzi F, Scotti G, di Natale B, et al. Evidence of a midline brain anomaly in pituitary dwarfs: a magnetic resonance imaging study in 101 patients. Pediatrics 1994;93:409–16.

37. Pampanini V, Pedicelli S, Gubinelli J, et al. Brain magnetic resonance imaging as first-line investigation for growth hormone deficiency diagnosis in early childhood. Horm Res Paediatr 2015;84:323–30.

38. Hamilton J, Blaser S, Danneman D. MR imaging in idiopathic growth hormone deficiency. Am J Neuroradiol 1998;19:1609–15.

39. Tauber M, Chevret J, Gwenaelle D, et al. Long-term evolution of endocrine disorders and effect of GH therapy in 35 patients with pituitary stalk interruption syndrome. Horm Res 2005;64:266–73.

40. Blum WF, Deal C, Zimmerman AG, et al. Development of additional pituitary hormone deficiencies in pediatric patients originally diagnosed with idiopathic isolated GH deficiency. Eur J Endocrinol 2014;170:13–21.

41. Fang C, George AS, Brinkmeier M, et al. Genetics of combined pituitary hormone deficiency: roadmap into the genome era. Endocr Rev 2016;37:636–75.

42. Kelberman D, Dattani MT. Genetics of septo-optic dysplasia. Pituitary 2007;10: 393–407.

43. Roessler E, Du YZ, Mullor JL, et al. Loss-of-function mutations in the human GLI2 gene are associated with pituitary anomalies and holoprosencephaly-like features. Proc Natl Acad Sci U S A 2003;100:13424–9.

44. Pai KG, Rubin HM, Wedemeyer PP, et al. Hypothalamic-pituitary dysfunction following group B beta hemolytic streptococcal meningitis in a neonate. J Pediatr 1978;88:289–91.

45. Saranac L, Bjelaovic B, Djordyevic D, et al. Hypopituitarism occurring in neonatal sepsis. J Pediatr Endocrinol Metab 2012;25:847–8.

46. Miller WL, Kaplan SL, Grumbach MM. Child abuse as a cause of post-traumatic hypopituitarism. N Engl J Med 1980;302:724–8.

47. Rona RJ, Tanner JM. Aetiology of idiopathic growth hormone deficiency in England and Wales. Arch Dis Child 1977;52:197–208.

48. Craft WH, Underwood LE, Van Wyk JJ. High incidence of perinatal insult in children with idiopathic hypopituitarism. J Pediatr 1980;96:397–402.

49. Geysenbergh B, De Catte L, Vogels A. Can fetal ultrasound result in prenatal diagnosis of Prader-Willi syndrome? Genet Couns 2011;22:207–16.

50. Binder G, Martin DD, Kanther I, et al. The course of neonatal cholestasis in congenital combined pituitary hormone deficiency. J Pediatr Endocrinol Metab 2007;20:695–701.

51. Mauvais F-X, Gonzales E, Davit-Spraul A, et al. Cholestasis reveals severe cortisol deficiency in neonatal pituitary stalk interruption syndrome. PLoS One 2016;11(2):e0147550.

52. Grimberg A, DiVall SA, Polychronakos C, et al. Guidelines for growth hormone and insulin-like growth factor-I treatment in children and adolescents: growth hormone deficiency, idiopathic short stature, and primary insulin-like growth factor-I deficiency. Horm Res Paediatr 2016;86:361–97.

53. Di Lorghi N, Allegri AEM, Napoli F, et al. The use of neuroimaging for assessing disorders of pituitary development. Clin Endocrinol 2012;76:161–76.

54. Maghnie M, Genovese E, Villa A, et al. Dynamic MRI in congenital agenesis of the neural pituitary stalk; the role of the vascular pituitary stalk in predicting residual anterior pituitary function. Clin Endocinol (Oxf) 1996;45:281–90.

55. Tocchio S, Kline-Faith B, Kanal E, et al. MRI evaluation and safety in the developing brain. Semin Perinatol 2015;39:73–104.

56. Hawkes CP, Grimberg A. Measuring growth hormone and insulin-like growth factor-I in infants: what is normal? Pediatr Endocrinol Rev 2013;11:126–46.

57. Leger J, Noel M, Limal JM, et al. Growth factors and intrauterine growth retardation. II. Serum growth hormone, insulin-like growth factor-I, and IGF-binding protein 3 levels in children with intrauterine growth retardation compared with normal control subjects: prospective study from birth to two years of age. Pediatr Res 1996;40:101–7.

58. Vavarigou V, Vagenakis AG, Makri M, et al. Growth hormone, insulin-like growth factor-I and prolactin in small for gestational age newborns. Biol Neonate 1994;65:94–102.

59. Binder G, Weidenkeller M, Blumenstock G, et al. Rational approach to the diagnosis of severe growth hormone deficiency in the newborn. J Clin Endocrinol Metab 2010;95:2219–26.

60. Binder G, Hettmann S, Weber K, et al. Analysis of the GH content within archived dried blood spots of newborn screening cards from children diagnosed with growth hormone deficiency after the neonatal period. Growth Horm IGF Res 2011;21:314–7.

61. Kelly A, Tang R, Becker S, et al. Poor specificity of low growth hormone and cortisol levels during fasting hypoglycemia for the diagnoses of growth hormone deficiency and adrenal insufficiency. Pediatrics 2008;122:E522–8.

62. Senniappan S, Hussain K. An evaluation of growth hormone and IGF-I responses in neonates with hyperinsulinemic hypoglycemia. Int J Endocrinol 2013;2013: 638257.

63. Mehta A, Hindmarsh PC, Dattani MT. An update on the biochemical diagnosis of congenital ACTH insufficiency. Clin Endocrinol 2005;62:307–14.

64. Maghnie M, Uga E, Temporini F, et al. Evaluation of adrenal function in patients with growth hormone deficiency and hypothalamic-pituitary disorders: comparison between insulin-induced hypoglycemia, low-dose ACTH, standard ACTH and CRH stimulation tests. Eur J Endocrinol 2005;152:735–41.

65. Grumbach MM. A window of opportunity: the diagnosis of gonadotropin deficiency in the male infant. J Clin Endocrinol Metab 2005;90:3122–7.

66. Braslavsky D, Grinspon RP, Ballerini MG, et al. Hypogonadotropic hypogonadism in infants with congenital hypopituitarism: a challenge to diagnose at an early stage. Horm Res Paediatr 2015;84:289–97.

67. Higuchi A, Hasegawa Y. Dose adjustments of hydrocortisone and L-thyroxine in hypopituitarism associated with cholestasis. Clin Pediatr Endocrinol 2006;15: 93–6.

Use of Glucocorticoids for the Fetus and Preterm Infant

Susan M. Scott, MD, JD[a],*, Susan R. Rose, MD, MEd[b]

KEYWORDS

- Glucocorticoids • HPA axis • Fetus • Newborn • BPD • Hypotension
- Brain development

KEY POINTS

- Glucocorticoids have positive short-term impact on preterm infant survival.
- The environment impacts glucocorticoids on brain development in the preterm infant.
- Fetal and preterm function of the HPA axis are immature, possibly linked also to thyroid hormone dysfunction.

Use of glucocorticoid (GC) treatment in the prenatal state and in the preterm infant has been evaluated for more than 40 years.[1] Many issues have been studied, including the following:

1. Historical use of GC therapy in the fetus and preterm infant.
2. Selection of which GCs have been used prenatally and postnatally.
3. Impact of GC treatment in the preterm infant. Are outcomes for the fetus and for postnatal development enhanced by use of GCs?
4. Role of GCs in the transition to postnatal life in full-term infants.

GC treatment in the fetus and preterm infant was demonstrated to be a highly successful therapeutic intervention resulting in decreasing occurrence of many consequences of preterm birth, at a time when ventilator dependence was a growing problem.[2] This outcome was based on giving GC 1 to 10 days before delivery, and not continuing to give the medication after birth. However, long-term negative effects were observed in subsequent studies of GC therapy, not necessarily predictable when use of dexamethasone began.[3]

Disclosure Statement: None.
[a] University of New Mexico School of Medicine, 2211 Lomas Boulevard, Albuquerque, NM 87131, USA; [b] Cincinnati Children's Hospital Medical Center and University of Cincinnati, MLC 7012, 3333 Burnet Avenue, Cincinnati, OH 45229, USA
* Corresponding author.
E-mail address: sscott@salud.unm.edu

Early interest in using exogenous GC included studies published in 1969 in prematurely delivered sheep that demonstrated improved outcome with GC therapy.[4] Of note, mean weight of the adrenal gland was 19% lighter in neonates dying of respiratory distress syndrome (RDS) within 72 hours of delivery, compared with adrenal weight in neonates who died of other causes.[5] Overall, results from sheep and humans suggested a role for GC in successful transition of the preterm infant to postnatal life. Betamethasone used predelivery in a controlled study was associated with a decrease in RSD occurrence in their infants.[6] However, despite many studies since then, there are still unresolved issues.[7,8]

Postnatal effects of GC therapy were noted in 1976 when women were given a single dose of hydrocortisone, 100 mg.[9] Infants born less than 24 hours after steroid therapy had no improved outcome. If the steroids were given greater than 24 hours before delivery, incidence and mortality associated with RDS were lowered. In addition, there was no acceleration of delivery, a concern because of a prior observation of increased contractions with GC infusion in the fetal state. It is unclear how the steroid dosage was chosen for these mothers. Lack of clarification of the rationale for choice of GC medication, dose, and duration of treatment are common issues in the literature. Several other studies during the same time period examined whether steroid therapy decreased occurrence of RDS.[10–12]

One of the reasons that GC therapy was initiated historically was the recognition of a poorly functioning fetal hypothalamic-pituitary-adrenal (HPA) axis in preterm infants. The fetus and placenta work together in controlling HPA axis action during pregnancy. Also controlled tightly during pregnancy are the types and levels of thyroid hormone encountered by the fetus. Then, as delivery approaches, changes in thyroid and cortisol concentrations begin to prepare the fetus for postnatal life.

The HPA axis does not function well early on after preterm delivery, especially when "stressed" or elevated levels of GCs are needed for successful postnatal transition of the preterm infant.[13,14] Even at 2 weeks of postnatal age, the corticotropin-releasing hormone (CRH) stimulation test (testing function of the pituitary) does not yield normal results in infants born at less than 30 weeks gestational age.[15]

Many studies have addressed suppression of the HPA axis by prenatal and/or postnatal GC treatment. Some of the results may be related to developmental delay in function of the HPA axis in the preterm infant. Replacement/treatment with GCs seems to be necessary for improved outcome in the preterm infant.[16]

The pattern of cortisol secretion after delivery depends on gestational age at birth. Ill infants born at greater than 27 weeks gestational age have rising cortisol values from Day 2 to Day 6, contrasted with cortisol values decreasing in well infants of the same age. Of note, a rise in cortisol is expected as a normal response to the physiologic stress of illness. In contrast, cortisol values significantly declined from Day 2 to Day 6 in well and ill infants who were born at less than or equal to 27 weeks gestational age. The cortisol concentrations in the premature infant are significantly correlated with gestational age and with markers of illness.[17] Postnatal effects after the use of antenatal steroids included a potential altered heart rate response to stressors later in life.[18]

TYPES OF GLUCOCORTICOIDS USED PRENATALLY

Unlike the preterm infant where several GCs have been used, there are two GCs that have been used primarily in the fetus: dexamethasone and betamethasone, often used at high doses. Both have been associated with subtly altered neurodevelopmental outcomes.[7]

Other GCs could be used, but the placenta does not inactivate dexamethasone and betamethasone. In contrast, hydrocortisone is metabolized by the placenta, so even though the shorter half-life of hydrocortisone (compared with dexamethasone and betamethasone) might result in fewer long-term negative effects, hydrocortisone might not have any recognizable effects in the fetus.[19]

In fetal congenital adrenal hyperplasia, dexamethasone crosses the placenta and suppresses expression of androgen-related steroids. This reduces exposure to androgen excess in female infants (including virilization of the genitalia), but also exposes male fetuses unnecessarily to GC. Concern about potential negative effects on brain development for all of these fetuses resulted in significant decrease in clinical use of early fetal dexamethasone for prevention of androgen exposure.[20]

TYPES OF GLUCOCORTICOIDS USED IN THE PRETERM INFANT

When GCs were first used in neonates, the choice of which to use was often based on excess water retention in the preterm newborn. The weight of the preterm newborn often did not decrease over time. Pure GC hormones could be used with no fluid retention. The rationale for dexamethasone use postnatally was that it has no mineralocorticoid effects.

Using a steroid with no mineralocorticoid effect, the newborn theoretically would lose more excess water and have a better outcome. However, although dexamethasone at replacement dosing is more of a pure GC than are other GCs, dexamethasone is a fluorinated GC. Fluorinated GC may be detrimental to brain development during childhood. In addition, the half-life of dexamethasone was unknown for preterm infants, compared with the known half-life for other GCs.

Dexamethasone, betamethasone, and hydrocortisone are the most common GCs used clinically in infants after premature delivery. More recently, inhaled GCs also have been studied, but have not consistently shown benefit in preterm infants with lung damage.[21–23] Negative outcomes have been less common with hydrocortisone treatment.[24]

Another issue in publications is how long a GC should be used to have benefit.[25] To mimic stressed release of GC in a setting of illness, only 5 days of dexamethasone was used after ventilator treatment (for more than 7 days) to evaluate whether GC could shorten the process of weaning preterm infants off the ventilator. Dexamethasone was effective in getting preterm infants (who had not previously received exogenous GC) off the ventilator faster.[25] However, peak cortisol response to the corticotropin hormone stimulation test was lower after dexamethasone therapy than after no steroid therapy. The reduced cortisol release was not clearly a result of GC therapy, because the extubated infant was under less stress.

POSITIVE BENEFITS OF GLUCOCORTICOIDS DURING PREGNANCY AND POSTNATALLY

Prenatal GC therapy has decreased the incidence of RDS, intraventricular hemorrhage, patent ductus arteriosus (PDA), and necrotizing enterocolitis in infants born preterm. Thus prenatal GC therapy continues to be used.[3,26] The most studied area of postnatal GC therapy has been in reduction of long-term lung damage, as is seen with bronchopulmonary dysplasia (see the algorithm at end of the article).[27]

NEGATIVE EFFECTS OF GLUCOCORTICOIDS USED DURING PREGNANCY AND POSTNATALLY

Concerns about potential negative effects of GC therapy have included effects on preterm uterine contractions, heart rate, brain development, and suppression of the HPA axis. Early in the study of GC treatment, a risk for premature uterine contractions was reported in sheep.[28] Over time, tocolytic methods were applied to prevent earlier delivery after use of GC. Also of concern was an apparent effect of GC on later life heart rate reactivity to stressors. The infants exposed to GC had high heart rates, and did not further increase heart rate under stress.[18]

The most studied negative impacts have included effects on neurologic development, and on suppression of the HPA axis. Issues of importance in delineating negative effects include the type of GC that is used, gestational age at which GC therapy is started, GC dosage, and duration of GC therapy. Few studies have been able to compare the types of GC. Fluorinated steroids, such as dexamethasone, have been noted to have more of a negative effect on brain function than does hydrocortisone.[29] Dexamethasone therapy has extended over a long period of time, such as 4 to 6 weeks. Even tapering the dose over a 6-week period continued suppression of the HPA axis for most of the 6-week period. Therefore, preterm infants were exposed to high-dose GC for many weeks.

Most studies of hydrocortisone therapy postnatally found a smaller or absent negative effect.[30–32] Use of GC can be associated with long-term effects on cognition, behavior, and memory (primarily through an impact on the hippocampus), particularly with the use of dexamethasone.[33] Dexamethasone was associated with worse outcome at 3 months of age than was use of hydrocortisone.[34] Regarding age of starting dexamethasone, beginning at 2 weeks of postnatal age presented more of a risk for poor outcome, than when started at 4 weeks.[35] Better outcomes for brain impact (in particular for brain volumes) are observed with hydrocortisone.[36,37] Dexamethasone given in infancy can have a negative effect persisting into the teenage years.[38]

Another issue is potential suppression of the HPA axis with exogenous use of GCs. Because the HPA axis is immature and often not functioning appropriately for postnatal life at time of delivery, interpretation of adrenocortical function tests is a challenge.[15,39–42] As with neurologic concerns, recovery of the HPA axis is easier to demonstrate in preterm infants given hydrocortisone. One study used a large dose of hydrocortisone in preterm infants born at less than 26 weeks gestation. Evaluation of response to the CRH test at 12 months of age showed that the HPA axis had recovered.[43] Thus, providing very early preterm infants with a daily low dose of hydrocortisone therapy does not lead to a serious suppressive effect on later function of the HPA axis.

Further articles on the impact of GC therapy have found minimal evidence of long-term cardiovascular effects[44] and transient reductions of cord blood growth hormone concentrations.[45] Prenatal GC therapy effects on 17-hydroxyprogesterone may interfere with newborn screening in identifying congenital adrenal hyperplasia.[46] Betamethasone use in preterm neonates reduced endogenous 17-OHP and cortisol levels, but had no effect on adrenal gland size.[46]

ROLE OF GLUCOCORTICOIDS IN TRANSITION

It has been recommended to use GC therapy for potential preterm delivery between 24 and 34 weeks gestation.[47] The rationale for using GC therapy has a great deal to do with understanding the role cortisol plays in successful transition of the fetus to postnatal life. In addition, GC therapy in the preterm fetus should mimic the impact of endogenous release of GC before delivery in the full-term infant.[8] A systematic review of randomized trials of perinatal GC therapy including more than 10,000 infants, compared outcomes in infants who received antenatal GC with outcomes in those receiving either placebo or no treatment. This review clearly demonstrated that GCs have a positive impact in reducing occurrence of RDS, severity of RDS, and even reducing the need for ventilation.[48]

Such evidence for GC therapy having benefits raises the issue of inherent developmental hormonal problems. Prenatal process of maturation seen for cortisol is similar to that seen for thyroid hormones. The systems "get ready to go," but the exposure of the fetus to these two hormones is regulated during prenatal life. Thyroid hormone and cortisol work together postnatally. In preparation for postnatal life, cortisol increase leads to an increase in T3 concentrations in the body.[49–51] Cortisol exerts influences on multiple organs in the perinatal period. It promotes fluid egress from the lung airways thereby enhancing the effect of surfactant. Moreover, GC may promote lung development in specific situations by reducing airway inflammation related to developmental immaturity, infection, or trauma. In contrast, lower circulating cortisol concentrations in the first week of life have been associated with adverse respiratory outcomes in preterm infants, a higher incidence of PDA, and increasing severity of lung inflammation.[52]

A second effect of cortisol is to thicken the skin by increasing the fat mass under the skin. This allows the infant to control loss of heat.[53] A third effect of cortisol is to prepare the kidneys for postnatal life. As has been demonstrated in the setting of hypopituitarism, normal renal free water clearance requires adequate exposure to cortisol. Preterm infants who were often described as being waterlogged because of inadequate diuresis benefited from prenatal steroid therapy with improved weight loss, increased urine output, and better lung function.[53] A fourth effect of cortisol is to prepare the gut for normal intestinal contractions. Preterm infants who do not tolerate oral nutrition may well be cortisol insufficient.[54]

A fifth effect is related to stability of blood pressure. Instability of blood pressure is a sign of cortisol insufficiency at any age. It is well known that treatment of hypotension solely with traditional pressers is not effective in a setting of hypocortisolism.[55–62] In several studies, hydrocortisone was used to treat low blood pressure and compared with the impact of dopamine. Overall, hydrocortisone is an appropriate therapy to use in the setting of a low corticotropin hormone stimulation test result suggesting adrenal insufficiency. Several studies have examined this issue in the preterm infant and in children and adults, using mainly hydrocortisone as treatment of refractory hypotension.

In summary, exogenous GCs have beneficial effects on occurrence of RDS and blood pressure alterations in the preterm infant.[63] Other more subtle issues include urine output, gastrointestinal responsiveness to feedings, and thickening of the skin. The outcome of greatest concern is the potential detrimental effect on brain development. However, this concern may be balanced by reduced morbidity and mortality of preterm birth after GC therapy.

Best Practices

What is the current practice?

- Guidelines suggest benefit from use of betamethasone before delivery for fetuses likely to be born between 24 and 34 weeks gestation (see algorithm).
- The American Academy of Pediatrics has stated that evidence is insufficient to recommend steroid therapy for all children with RDS. Studies of which medications, their dosing, and their length of use are required.

However,

- In the preterm infant, the use of GC therapy reduces the occurrence and severity of RDS.
- Use of hydrocortisone therapy is expected to cause fewer negative effects than the use of other steroids.

What changes in current practice are likely to improve outcomes?

- Prenatal use of betamethasone may result in better outcomes than use of dexamethasone.
- Dexamethasone crosses the placenta, but may have significant negative neurologic outcomes.
- Hydrocortisone does not cross the placenta.
- For the preterm infant, hydrocortisone is currently the most beneficial GC therapy being applied.

Major recommendations

For the prenatal state:
- Use of betamethasone in potential preterm delivery at less than or equal to 34 weeks gestation.
- Using GC as therapy for one or two treatments is recommended, but not to continue therapy.

For the preterm infant:
- There are no major recommendations.

Summary Statement

Overall, GC treatment has improved the outcome of the preterm infant.

Algorithm for Use of Prenatal Steroid Therapy (derived from Ref.[47])

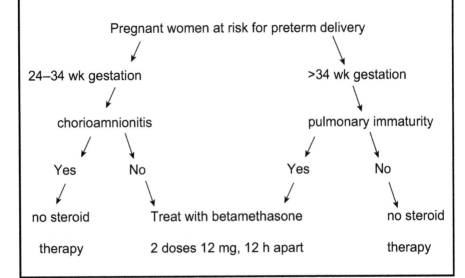

REFERENCES

1. Cottrell EC, Secki JR. Prenatal stress, glucocorticoids and the programming of adult disease. Front Behav Neurosci 2009;3(19):1–9.
2. Hallman M. The story of antenatal steroid therapy before preterm birth. Neonatology 2015;107:352–7.
3. Bartholomew J, Kovacs L, Papagerogiou A. Review of the antenatal and postnatal use of steroids. Indian J Pediatr 2014;81:466–72.
4. Liggins GC. Premature delivery of foetal lambs infused with glucocorticoids. J Endocrinol 1969;45:515.
5. Naeye RL, Harcke HT Jr, Blanc WA. Adrenal gland structure and the development of hyaline membrane disease. Pediatrics 1971;47:650–7.
6. Liggins GC, Howie RN. A controlled trial of antepartum glucocorticoid treatment for prevention of the respiratory distress syndrome in premature infants. Pediatrics 1972;50:515–25.
7. Waffarn F, Davis EP. Effects of antenatal corticosteroids on the hypothalamic-pituitary-adrenocortical axis of the fetus and newborn: experimental findings and clinical considerations. Am J Obstet Gynecol 2012;207:446–54.
8. Hillman NH, Kallapur SG, Jobe AH. Physiology of transition from intrauterine to extrauterine life. Clin Perinatol 2012;39:769–83.
9. Dluholucky S, Babic J, Taufer I. Reduction of incidence and mortality of respiratory distress syndrome by administration of hydrocortisone to mother. Arch Dis Child 1976;51:420–3.
10. Morrison JC, Whybrew WD, Bucovaz ET, et al. Injection of corticosteroids into mother to prevent neonatal respiratory distress syndrome. Am J Obstet Gynecol 1978;131:358–66.
11. Gluck L. Administration of corticosteroids to induce maturation of fetal lung. Am J Dis Child 1976;130:976–8.
12. Ballard RA, Ballard PL. Use of prenatal glucocorticoid therapy to prevent respiratory distress syndrome. A supporting view. Am J Dis Child 1976;130:982–7.
13. Nykänen P, Anttila E, Heinonen K, et al. Early hypoadrenalism in premature infants at risk for bronchopulmonary dysplasia or death. Acta Paediatr 2007;96:1600–5.
14. Bolt RJ, Van Weissenbruch MM, Popp-Snijders C, et al. Maturity of the adrenal cortex in very preterm infants is related to gestational age. Pediatr Res 2002;52:405–10.
15. Niwa F, Kawai M, Kanazawa H, et al. Limited response to CRH stimulation tests at 2 weeks of age in preterm infants born at less than 30 weeks of gestational age. Clin Endocrinol (Oxf) 2013;78:724–9.
16. Fernandez EF, Watterberg KL. Relative adrenal insufficiency in the preterm and term infant. J Perinatol 2009;29(Suppl 2):S44–9.
17. Scott SM, Watterberg KL. Effect of gestational age, postnatal age, and illness on cortisol concentrations in premature infants. Pediatr Res 1995;37:112–6.
18. Weiss SJ, Niemann S. Effects of antenatal corticosteroids on cortisol and heart rate reactivity of preterm infants. Biol Res Nurs 2015;17:487–94.
19. Lekarev O, New MI. Adrenal disease in pregnancy. Best Pract Res Clin Endocrinol Metab 2011;25:959–73.
20. Miller WL, Witchel SF. Prenatal treatment of congenital adrenal hyperplasia: risks outweigh benefits. Am J Obstet Gynecol 2013;208:354–9.
21. Koch A, Kreutzer K, von Oldershausen G, et al, NEuroSIS Trial Group. Inhaled glucocorticoids and pneumonia in preterm infants: post hoc result from the NEurosSIS Trial. Neonatology 2017;29:110–3.

22. Bassler D, Plavka R, Shinwell ES, et al, NEUROSIS Trail Group. Early inhaled budesonide for the prevention of bronchopulmonary dysplasia. N Engl J Med 2015; 373:1497–506.

23. Bassler D. Inhalation or instillation of steroids for the prevention of bronchopulmonary dysplasia. Neonatology 2015;107:358–9.

24. Peltoniemi OM, Lano A, Puosi R, et al, Neonatal Hydrocortisone Working Group. Trial of early neonatal hydrocortisone: two-year follow-up. Neonatology 2009;95: 240–7.

25. Scott SM, Backstrom C, Bessman S. Effects of five days of dexamethasone therapy on ventilator dependence and adrenacorticotropic hormone-stimulated cortisol concentrations. J Perinatol 1997;17:24–8.

26. Fowden AL, Juan L, Forhead AJ. Glucocorticoids and the preparation for life after birth: are there long-term consequences of the life insurance? Proc Nutr Soc 1998;57:113–22.

27. Baud O, Maury L, Lebail F, et al, PREMILOC trial study group. Effect of early low-dose hydrocortisone on survival without bronchopulmonary dysplasia in extremely preterm infants (PREMILOC): a double-blind, placebo-controlled, multicentre, randomised trial. Lancet 2016;387:1827–36.

28. Liggins GC, Grieves SA, Kendall JZ, et al. The physiological roles of progesterone, oestradiol-17B and prostaglandin F2-a in the control of ovine parturition. J Reprod Fertil 1972;16(Suppl 16):85.

29. Baud O. Postnatal steroid treatment and brain development. Arch Dis Child Fetal Neonatal Ed 2004;89:F96–100.

30. Needelman H, Hoskoppal A, Roberts H, et al. The effect of hydrocortisone on neurodevelopmental outcome in premature infants less than 29 weeks' gestation. J Child Neurol 2010;25:448–52.

31. Rademaker KJ, Uiterwaal CS, Groenendaal F, et al. Neonatal hydrocortisone treatment: neurodevelopmental outcome and MRI at school age in preterm-born children. J Pediatr 2007;150:351–7.

32. Parikh NA, Kennedy KA, Lasky RE, et al. Neurodevelopmental outcomes of extremely preterm infants randomized to stress dose hydrocortisone. PLoS One 2015;10:e0137051.

33. Change YP. Evidence for adverse effect of perinatal glucocorticoid use on the developing brain. Korean J Pediatr 2014;57:101–9.

34. Hitzert MM, Benders MJ, Roescher AM, et al. Hydrocortisone vs. dexamethasone treatment for bronchopulmonary dysplasia and their effects on general movements in preterm infants. Pediatr Res 2012;7:100–6.

35. Papile LA, Tyson JE, Stoll BJ, et al. Multi-center trial of two dexamethasone regimens in ventilator-dependent premature infants. N Engl J Med 1998;338:1112–8.

36. Kersbergen KJ, de Vries LS, van Kooij BJ, et al. Hydrocortisone treatment for bronchopulmonary dysplasia and brain volumes in preterm infants. J Pediatr 2013;163:666–71.

37. Parikh NA, Kennedy KA, Lasky RE, et al. Pilot randomized trial of hydrocortisone in ventilator-dependent extremely preterm infants: effects on regional brain volumes. J Pediatr 2013;162:685–90.e1.

38. ter Wolbeek M, de Sonneville LM, de Vries WB, et al. Early life intervention with glucocorticoids has negative effects on motor development and neuropsychological function in 14-17 year-old adolescents. Psychoneuroendocrinology 2013;38: 975–86.

39. Watterberg KL, Scott SM. Evidence of early adrenal insufficiency in babies who develop bronchopulmonary dysplasia. Pediatr 1995;95:120–5.

40. Walther FJ, Findlay RD, Durand M. Adrenal suppression and extubation rate after moderately early low-dose dexamethasone therapy in very preterm infants. Early Hum Dev 2003;74:37–45.
41. Ng PC, Lam CW, Lee CH, et al. Suppression and recovery of the hypothalamic function after high-dose corticosteroid treatment in preterm infants. Neonatology 2008;94:170–5.
42. Battin MR, Bevan C, Harding JE. Repeat doses of antenatal steroids and hypothalamic-pituitary-adrenal axis (HPA) function. Am J Obstet Gynecol 2007; 197:40.e1-6.
43. Takayanagi T, Matsuo K, Egashira T, et al. Neonatal hydrocortisone therapy does not have a serious suppressive effect on the later function of the hypothalamus-pituitary-adrenal axis. Acta Paediatr 2015;104:e195–9.
44. McKinlay CJ, Cutfield WS, Battin MR, et al, ACTORDS Study Group. Cardiovascular risk factors in children after repeat doses of antenatal glucocorticoids: an RCT. Pediatrics 2015;135:e405–15.
45. Ballard PL, Gluckman PD, Liggins GC, et al. Steroid and growth hormone levels in preterm infants after prenatal betamethasone therapy to prevent respiratory distress syndrome. Pediatr Res 1980;14:122–7.
46. Buyukkayhan D, Ozturk MA, Kurtoglu S, et al. Effect of antenatal betamethasone use on adrenal gland size and endogenous cortisol and 17-hydroxyprogesterone in preterm neonates. J Pediatr Endocrinol Metab 2009;22:1027–41.
47. Watterberg KL. Committee on fetus and newborn. Postnatal corticosteroids to prevent or treat bronchopulmonary dysplasia. Pediatr 2010;126:800–8.
48. Roberts D, Brown J, Medley N, et al. Antenatal corticosteroids for accelerating fetal lung maturation for women at risk of preterm birth. Cochrane Database Syst Rev 2017;(3):CD004454.
49. Yagasaki H, Kobayashi K, Nemoto A, et al. Late-onset circulatory dysfunction after thyroid hormone treatment in an extremely low birth weight infant. J Pediatr Endocrinol Metab 2010;23:153–8.
50. Ballard PL. Hormonal influences during fetal lung development. Ciba Found Symp 1980;78:251–74.
51. Scott SM, Cimino DF. Evidence for developmental hypopituitarism in ill preterm infants. J Perinatol 2004;24:429–34.
52. Watterberg KL, Scott SM, Backstrom C, et al. Links between early adrenal function and respiratory outcome in preterm infants: airway inflammation and patent ductus arteriosus. Pediatr 2000;105:320–4.
53. Dimitriou G, Kavvadia V, Marcou M, et al. Antenatal steroids and fluid balance in very low birthweight infants. Arch Dis Child Fetal Neonatal Ed 2005;90:F509–13.
54. Costalos C, Gounaris A, Sevastiadou S, et al. The effect of antenatal corticosteroids on gut peptides of preterm infants-a matched group comparison: corticosteroids and gut development. Early Hum Dev 2003;74:83–8.
55. Fernandez E, Schrader R, Watterberg K. Prevalence of low cortisol values in term and near-term infants with vasopressor-resistant hypotension. J Perinatol 2005; 25:114–8.
56. Salas G, Travaglianti M, Leone A, et al. Hydrocortisone for the treatment of refractory hypotension: a randomized controlled trial. An Pediatr (Barc) 2014;80: 387–93.
57. Hochwald O, Palegra G, Osiovich H. Adding hydrocortisone as 1st line of inotropic treatment for hypotension in very low birth weight infants. Indian J Pediatr 2014;81:808–10.

58. Mizobuchi M, Yoshimoto S, Nakao H. Time-course effect of a single dose of hydrocortisone for refractory hypotension in preterm infants. Pediatr Int 2011;53: 881–6.

59. Higgins S, Friedlich P, Seri I. Hydrocortisone for hypotension and vasopressor dependence in preterm neonates: a meta-analysis. J Perinatol 2010;30:373–8.

60. Baker CF, Barks JD, Engmann C, et al. Hydrocortisone administration for the treatment of refractory hypotension in critically ill newborns. J Perinatol 2008; 28:412–9.

61. Seri I. Hydrocortisone and vasopressor-resistant shock in preterm neonates. Pediatr 2006;117:516–8.

62. Ng PC, Lee CH, Lam CW, et al. Transient adrenocortical insufficiency of prematurity and systemic hypotension in very low birthweight infants. Arch Dis Child Fetal Neonatal Ed 2004;89:F119–26.

63. Miracle X, DiRenzo GC, Stark A, et al. Guideline for the use of antenatal corticosteroids for fetal maturation. J Perinat Med 2008;36:191–6.

Neonatal Cushing Syndrome

A Rare but Potentially Devastating Disease

Christina Tatsi, MD, PhD[a,b],
Constantine A. Stratakis, MD, D(Med)Sc[a,b],*

KEYWORDS

- Cushing syndrome • Hypercortisolemia • Adrenocortical tumors
- Adrenal hyperplasia • Infant

KEY POINTS

- Neonatal Cushing syndrome (CS) is a rare disorder, but it can lead to significant complications and even death, if not diagnosed and treated promptly.
- Adrenocortical tumors (ACTs) are a common cause of neonatal CS and they can be adrenocortical carcinomas.
- Neonatal CS may present as part of a genetic syndrome, such as Li-Fraumeni syndrome, McCune-Albright syndrome, Beckwith-Wiedemann syndrome, and DICER1 mutations.
- Diagnosis includes documentation of loss of the circadian rhythm of cortisol production (after it has been established), elevation of urinary free cortisol, and lack of suppression of cortisol production after dexamethasone administration.
- Surgical resection of the adrenal tumor is the current approach of treatment for ACTs. Adjuvant chemotherapy should be considered in cases of adrenocortical carcinomas.

INTRODUCTION

Cushing syndrome (CS) is named after Dr Harvey Cushing, an American neurosurgeon who first described the condition in a patient with weight gain, round face, hypertrichosis, muscle weakness, and irregular menstruations in 1912.[1] The term CS is currently

Disclosure Statement: The authors of this article declare that they have nothing to disclose.
[a] Section on Endocrinology and Genetics, Developmental Endocrine Oncology and Genetics Group, *Eunice Kennedy Shriver* National Institute of Child Health and Human Development (NICHD), National Institutes of Health (NIH), NIH-Clinical Research Center, 10 Center Drive, Building 10, Room 1-3330, MSC1103, Bethesda, MD 20892, USA; [b] Pediatric Endocrinology Inter-Institute Training Program, *Eunice Kennedy Shriver* National Institute of Child Health and Human Development (NICHD), National Institutes of Health (NIH), NIH-Clinical Research Center, 10 Center Drive, Building 10, Room 1-3330, MSC1103, Bethesda, MD 20892, USA
* Corresponding author. Section on Endocrinology and Genetics, Developmental Endocrine Oncology and Genetics Group, Eunice Kennedy Shriver National Institute of Child Health and Human Development, National Institutes of Health, NIH-Clinical Research Center, 10 Center Drive, Building 10, Room 1-3330, MSC1103, Bethesda, MD 20892.
E-mail address: stratakc@mail.nih.gov

Clin Perinatol 45 (2018) 103–118
https://doi.org/10.1016/j.clp.2017.10.002
0095-5108/18/Published by Elsevier Inc.

used to describe the constellation of signs and symptoms that result from the chronic effects of hypercortisolemia.[2]

The etiology of CS is divided into exogenous (or iatrogenic) CS and endogenous (adrenocorticotropic hormone [ACTH]-dependent and ACTH-independent) CS. The widespread use of glucocorticoid (GC) treatment for various conditions (autoimmune, malignant, allergic) has rendered exogenous CS a common condition.[3,4] The endogenous type is much more rare, with an estimated incidence of 2 to 5 new cases per million people diagnosed every year; of these, only 10% refer to children. Endogenous neonatal CS is extremely rare. Most of the cases present as part of an isolated adrenocortical tumor (ACT), often an adrenocortical carcinoma. Nearly 100 patients with neonatal and infantile CS not associated with isolated ACTs have been described to date (Supplemental Table 1).[5]

CS is associated with significant clinical findings, such as hypertension, hyperglycemia, hyperlipidemia, decreased bone mineral density, and muscular atrophy. More characteristically in children, CS also leads to growth arrest, despite continuous weight gain.[5] Given the severity of the various comorbidities, which may result in long-term and irreversible complications, it is essential to recognize and appropriately manage CS as soon as possible in any age, but particularly in infancy.

THE FETAL AND NEONATAL HYPOTHALAMIC–PITUITARY–ADRENAL AXIS

The adrenal glands derive from the urogenital ridge of the intermediate mesoderm, which also differentiates into the gonads and the mesonephros.[6,7] The development of the steroid-producing cells starts at 4 weeks of gestation, and at 5 weeks the adrenal cells are clearly separated from the gonads.[8] Around the same period (7 weeks of gestation), sympathetic nerve cells from the neural crest migrate to the center of the adrenals to form the adrenal medulla.[6] At 8 weeks of gestation, adrenals are distinct organs and the adrenal cortex consists of 2 separate zones, the fetal and the definitive zone.[9,10]

The fetal zone comprises almost 80% of the adrenal gland volume at term and it is a hormonally active region. However, it has low levels of 3-beta hydroxysteroid dehydrogenase and high levels of sulfotransferase enzyme concentrations, which renders dehydroepiandrosterone and dehydroepiandrosterone sulfate (DHEAS) the main product of the fetal zone.[11] Those substances are further used by the placenta to maintain the estriol levels.[12]

The fetal zone starts to involute after birth and disappears by the end of the first year of life.[10] The definitive zone, the outer zone that surrounds the fetal cortex, increases in size with age and it gives rise to the 3 known zones of the adult adrenal cortex (glomerulosa, fasciculata, and reticularis) within the first 1 to 3 years of life; development of zone reticularis is not completed until the puberty years.[13]

Cortisol has been detected as early as 8 weeks of gestation, and it has significant functions during the intrauterine life, including for the maturation of lungs, liver, thyroid, and other organs.[14] The human fetal adrenal gland starts also secreting aldosterone, desoxycorticosterone, and corticosterone between 10 and 20 weeks.[10] As mentioned, DHEAS levels are high at birth but decrease rapidly afterward as the fetal zone involutes.[10]

The adrenal production of cortisol is under the control of the HPA axis. Corticotropin-releasing hormone (CRH) production has been reported in primates by the third trimester.[15] However, sources of CRH production outside the hypothalamus, such as the placenta, have also been documented to contribute significantly in the cortisol production during embryogenesis.[16] The anterior lobe of the pituitary, where ACTH hormone is produced, derives from the oral ectoderm and it is fully formed by 5 weeks of gestation. Although ACTH is detected in the fetal pituitary by the 7th week of gestational age, its trophic properties become important for the maintenance of the fetal zone of the adrenals only after the first 4 to 5 months of gestation.[6,9] After birth, ACTH is the sole significant trophic factor of the definitive zone as the fetal zone gradually involutes.

CRH is synthesized in the hypothalamus and carried to the anterior pituitary in the portal system; this may first happen after the second trimester in fetal life. CRH stimulates ACTH release from the anterior pituitary, which in turn stimulates the adrenal cortex to secrete cortisol.[17,18] Cortisol further inhibits the synthesis and secretion of both CRH and ACTH in a negative feedback regulation system (**Fig. 1**). In children and adults (but not before 3–6 months of age), the hormones of the HPA axis follow a circadian rhythm of secretion. ACTH reaches a peak level between 06:00 to 08:00 hours, and a nadir level at 23:00 to 01:00 hours.[19] Similarly, cortisol levels peak some time between 07:30 and 08:30 hours and then decrease with a nadir value at midnight.[20]

The understanding of the physiology of the HPA axis is very important for the diagnostic workup of patients with CS, where autonomous secretion of ACTH and/or cortisol does not comply with these rules.

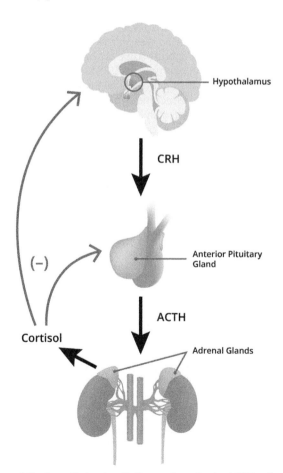

Fig. 1. Illustration of the hypothalamic–pituitary–adrenal axis. ACTH, adrenocorticotrophic hormone; CRH, corticotropin-releasing hormone.

CAUSES OF CUSHING SYNDROME
Exogenous Cushing Syndrome

The most commonly encountered cause of neonatal CS is the exogenous administration of pharmacologic doses of GCs, which comprises more than 95% of all cases. Although the report of the long-term complications of neonatal exposure to GCs (mainly metabolic and central nervous system related) has placed their perinatal use under consideration, GCs remain part of various therapeutic approaches, such as the management of fetal lung maturation prenatally, as well as respiratory, neurologic, and other conditions postnatally.[21–24] The effects of GCs on the suppression of the HPA is seen not only in systemic administration of the medications, but also in topically applied GCs.[25]

Endogenous Cushing Syndrome

The causes of endogenous CS are divided into ACTH-dependent and ACTH-independent (**Table 1**). Adrenal disorders cause ACTH-independent CS and they are the commonest cause of endogenous CS in neonates and infants. This category is very diverse, involving various adrenal diseases.

ACTs represent 0.2% of all pediatric tumors and they constitute the commonest cause of adrenal-dependent CS in the first years of life.[5,26] Although not all ACTs are associated with CS, signs of hypercortisolemia, isolated or in combination with hyperandrogenemia, have been identified in up to 50% of ACT cases.[27,28] ACTs are commonly malignant adrenocortical carcinoma with a poor prognosis (70% of cases), but they may also represent benign unilateral adrenocortical adenomas.[27] ACTs present at a median age of 3 to 4 years old, but cases present even at birth have been described.[27,28]

More rarely, benign bilateral adrenocorticortical hyperplasia may result in autonomous, ACTH-independent hypercortisolemia. This category is further divided according to the size of the nodules into macronodular (>1 cm) and micronodular (<1 cm) disease.[29,30] The micronodular adrenocortical nodular disease can be secondary to primary pigmented adrenocortical nodular disease (PPNAD) or nonpigmented isolated micronodular adrenocortical disease. In contrast, macronodular hyperplasia may present with multiple bilateral cortisol secreting nodules with internodular atrophy (bilateral macroadenomatous hyperplasia) or without atrophy (massive macronodular adrenal hyperplasia).[29,30]

Table 1 Causes of neonatal Cushing syndrome	
Cause	**Mechanism**
Exogenous	Iatrogenic administration of pharmacologic doses of GCs
ACTH-Dependent CS	Pituitary ACTH secreting adenoma (Cushing disease) Ectopic ACTH and/or CRH secretion Pituitary blastoma
ACTH-Independent CS	Adrenocortical carcinoma Adrenocortical adenoma Bilateral adrenocortical hyperplasias • Micronodular (size of nodules <1 cm) ○ Primary pigmented adrenocortical nodular disease ○ Isolated micronodular adrenocortical disease • Macronodular (size of nodules >1 cm) ○ Bilateral macroadenomatous hyperplasia ○ Massive macronodular adrenal hyperplasia

Abbreviations: ACTH, adrenocorticotrophic hormone; CRH, corticotropin-releasing hormone; CS, Cushing syndrome; GCs, glucocorticoids.

In older children and adults, ACTH-dependent CS results usually from pituitary corticotropin-secreting adenomas (this is known as Cushing disease [CD]).[2] The pituitary adenomas are commonly microadenomas (size of <1 cm) and more rare macroadenomas (size of >1 cm) that exhibit a semiautonomous secretion of ACTH, which further leads to bilateral adrenal stimulation and cortisol production.[31,32] Although CD is the commonest cause of CS in older children, its prevalence declines under the age of 7 years.[5,33] Recently, many of the previously reported infantile ACTH-secreting pituitary adenomas have been reclassified as pituitary blastomas.[34] These tumors are considered embryonal tumors, containing cells from all the stages of pituitary development as well as epithelial Rathke cells, which is a unique feature. In most of the reported cases, ACTH-dependent hypercortisolemia has been reported, but additional pituitary hormones might be oversecreted as well.[35]

On rare occasions, ACTH-dependent CS may result from ectopic ACTH and/or CRH production, where the source of the ectopic hormone production is located in the lungs, the liver, the thymus, the pancreas, or other neuroendocrine tumors.[36] In infancy specifically, reports of ectopic ACTH production from neuroblastomas represent the majority of ectopic CS.[37]

GENETIC CAUSES OF NEONATAL AND INFANTILE CUSHING SYNDROME

Various genetic causes have been associated with the pathogenesis of adrenal CS, both in the adult and the pediatric populations. *TP53* gene mutations are the most common cause of ACTs and are identified in almost 70% of ACTs.[38,39] This percentage is higher in pediatric patients with ACTs from Southern Brazil, where a point mutation of *TP53* gene (Arg337His) has been reported in 78% to 97% of cases.[40,41] Germline *TP53* gene mutations may cause Li-Fraumeni syndrome, which is an autosomal-dominant inherited syndrome predisposing to various cancers.[42] Patients with Li-Fraumeni syndrome present with early onset (childhood) ACTs and an increased risk for other malignancies (osteosarcoma, soft tissue sarcoma, breast cancer, brain tumors, leukemia, and others).[43] The penetrance of the germline mutations is variable and it has been suggested that any child with ACT should be assessed for *TP53* mutations, irrespective of the family history.[39]

Defects of various steps of the cyclic adenosine monophosphate–protein kinase A pathway have been also implicated in the pathogenesis of adrenal causes of CS.[33,38] McCune–Albright syndrome (MAS) presents with the clinical triad of bone fibrous dysplasia, café-au-lait macules, and precocious puberty. MAS results from postzygotic somatic mutations of the *GNAS* gene, which codes for the Gsa subunit of the G-protein–coupled receptors, causing their constitutive activation, which leads to increased levels of the intracellular cyclic adenosine monophosphate, irrespective of the ligand concentration.[44] Given the fact that many of the hormone receptors are G-coupled protein receptors, MAS may manifest as activating endocrinopathies of various types (hyperthyroidism, growth hormone excess, precocious puberty, and others).[44] The presence of CS in MAS has been described as early as in the neonatal period and it is uncommon after the first year of life.[45] It presents as either unilateral adrenal nodules or bilateral adenomata and/or hyperplasia.[46] The course of the disease is usually severe, even leading to death, but contrary to other CS cases, the patients who survive the acute phase of the disease without requiring adrenalectomy might experience spontaneous resolution.[45]

Additional defects of the cyclic adenosine monophosphate/protein kinase A pathway include mutations in the *PRKAR1A* gene, which codes for the regulatory subunit R1a of the protein kinase A, and are the leading cause of Carney complex.[47] Carney complex describes the association of myxomas, spotty skin pigmentation, endocrine overactivity, and psammomatous melanotic schwannomas. Up to 30% of patients with Carney complex present with PPNAD, some of them as children; however, no patient with PPNAD has ever been diagnosed with CS before the age of 1 year.[48] This may point to the different developmental origin of the adrenal lesions in PPNAD compared with other ACTs and MAS that present with CS in infancy.

Defects of the 11p15 locus involving *IGF2*, *H9*, and *CDKI* genes, either in the somatic state in the adrenal tumors or identified as germline defects, as in patients with Beckwith-Wiedemann syndrome (BWS), have also been associated with the presence of adrenal-dependent CS in the neonatal period.[49] BWS is a genetic overgrowth and cancer predisposition syndrome characterized by hemihypertrophy, macrosomia, macroglossia, organomegaly, hyperinsulinism, omphalocele/umbilical hernia, and distinct facial features.[50] Patients with BWS have an increased risk of developing intrabdominal tumors, including hepatoblastomas, Wilm's tumors, rhabdomyosarcomas, and ACTs, which are commonly identified early in life.[51] Although most of the ACTs are not resulting in CS, cases of hypercortisolemia have been reported in a few patients. CS in BWS may present as bilateral adrenal hyperplasia and it has been postulated to result from the delay of the maturation of the fetal adrenal gland.[52] More recently, an ACTH-secreting pituitary adenoma has been reported in a 17-year-old patient with BWS and CD; however, this is an infrequent presentation of the syndrome.[53]

Other genetic defects that cause ACTs and CS, include *MEN1* gene mutations causing multiple endocrine neoplasia type 1 (MEN1), *APC* gene defects causing familial adenomatous polyposis, and others such as *SF1*, *PRKACA, PDE11A, PDE8B*, and *ARMC5* genetic changes. However, none of these conditions are known to cause CS in infancy, and they are rarely the cause of hypercortisolemia before the age of 10 years.[33,54,55]

The genetic background of CD in children has been largely unknown until recently. Some of the known genes implicated in pituitary tumors, such as *MEN1, AIP, PRKAR1A, CDK1B*, and *CDKN2C*, explained only a small percentage of the pediatric cases.[56] Recently, Reincke and colleagues[57] reported a high frequency of somatic mutations of the *USP8* gene, which has also been confirmed in 31% of pediatric CD.[58] However, CD secondary to pituitary adenomas is rare in infants.

In contrast, pituitary blastomas appear to be present in most of the known cases of ACTH-dependent CS in infancy and most of these patients present with a germline or somatic *DICER1* gene mutation.[34] The DICER1 protein is a small RNA processing endoribonuclease that cleaves precursor microRNAs into mature microRNAs. Germline mutations of the *DICER1* gene cause the pleuropulmonary blastoma familial tumor and dysplasia syndrome, which involves the presence of multiple benign and malignant tumors in addition to pituitary blastomas.[59]

CLINICAL MANIFESTATIONS OF CUSHING SYNDROME

The clinical presentation of CS can be rather insidious and initially the signs may easily be confused with other more common entities, such as obesity or constitutional delay of growth.[30] However, as hypercortisolemia persists, the typical Cushingoid findings develop: central obesity, posterior neck fat deposition (buffalo hump), round facies, facial plethora, hirsutism, easy bruising, acne, and decreased bone mineral density **(Fig. 2, Table 2)**.[60–62] Certain Cushing-related manifestations, such as the violaceous striae, have been suggested to be less common in the infant population.[5,27]

In the growing infant and child specifically, one of the most important and earlier signs of isolated CS is the height deceleration along with continuous weight gain, which can be easily identified with review of the patient's growth chart.[63] Given, however, the high incidence of ACTs that co-secrete cortisol and androgens, an accelerated growth velocity has

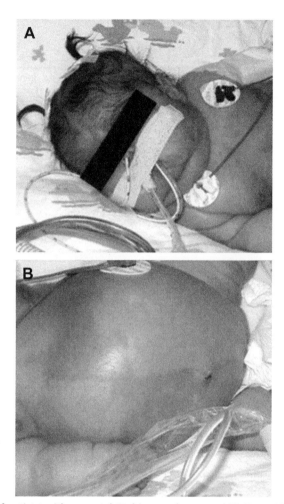

Fig. 2. Picture of patient with neonatal Cushing syndrome and McCune–Albright syndrome (MAS). Note the round cushingoid face, the body obesity, the hypertrichosis of the face (*A*) and the characteristic café-au-lait macules on the abdomen that respect the midline (*B*).

also been reported in 15% to 29% of these patients, and thus the absence of height deceleration cannot rule out the presence of hypercortisolemia. Furthermore, signs of hyperandrogenemia, including the presence of pubic hair, hypertrophy of the clitoris or the penis, acne, and hirsutism, may sometimes be the presenting finding.[27,28]

Hypercortisolemia may also induce suppression of the immune system and increased risk for severe and/or opportunistic infections. This is usually depicted on the abnormal white blood cell counts (leukocytosis, neutrophilia, and lymphopenia), whereas clinical cases of severe infections and even death secondary to cortisol induced immunosuppression have been reported.[64,65] Additional findings that are consequences of the hypercortisolemia include hypokalemia, hypercalcemia and hyperglycemia, although hypernatremia is less common.[60,66] Hypertension is a significant finding in the pediatric CS population because it can be difficult to manage.[67] Patients with hypertensive complications such as seizures, intracerebral hemorrhage, and hypertensive crisis, leading even to death, have been described previously.[27,68,69]

Table 2
Manifestations of neonatal Cushing syndrome

System	Finding
Growth	Obesity/weight gain
	Height deceleration
Skin	Easy bruising
	Striae
	Hirsutism
	Acne
	Dorsal fat pad
	Facial plethora
	Acanthosis nigricans
Cardiovascular	Hypertension
Musculoskeletal	Osteopenia and increased fracture risk
	Proximal muscle weakness
Immunologic	Lymphopenia
	Increased risk for infections
Neurocognitive	Sleep disorders
	Anxiety
	Depression
Abnormal laboratory findings	Hyperglycemia
	Hypokalemia
	Hyperlipidemia

DIAGNOSTIC APPROACH TO NEONATAL CUSHING SYNDROME

Although iatrogenic CS can easily be delineated by the review of the medical history of the patient and his previous and current medications, the diagnostic workup for endogenous CS involves various additional steps (**Fig. 3**).

The establishment of the diagnosis of hypercortisolemia is usually based on 3 criteria: (1) the loss of the circadian rhythm of the cortisol secretion as documented with an elevated midnight serum or salivary cortisol level, (2) the elevation of the 24-hour urine free cortisol, and (3) the lack of suppression of cortisol production after the administration of low-dose overnight dexamethasone (1 mg or equivalent weight-based dose of 15 μg/kg in children). The presence of 2 abnormal test results strongly supports the diagnosis of CS.[70] The completion of these tests can be complicated by the fact that the circadian rhythm of the neonates and infants does not necessarily follow the regular day/night rhythm of older children and adults. Circadian rhythms are just being established between 3 and 6 months of age. Additionally, the 24-hour urine collection can be uncomfortable to obtain, because the presence of an indwelling catheter is usually necessary. Thus, the interpretation of these tests should be done in conjunction with the clinical presentation of the patient.

Biochemical evaluation should also include the measurement of the adrenal androgens to identify the cases of GC and androgen co-secretion by adrenal tumors. DHEAS is the most specific adrenal hormone, because the enzyme sulfatase that converts dehydroepiandrosterone to DHEAS is found almost exclusively in the adrenals and 95% of the circulating DHEAS is coming from the adrenals. Additional hormones to be measured include androstenedione, testosterone, and estradiol. Other markers of accelerated cell turnover, such as lactate dehydrogenase, as well as tumor markers, such as alpha-fetoprotein, carcinoembryonic antigen, and cancer antigen 125, should also be sent as part of the evaluation before the surgery and they can

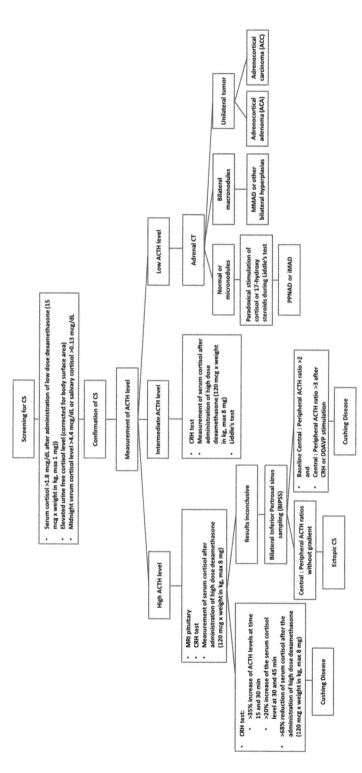

Fig. 3. Diagnostic approach to Cushing syndrome (CS). ACTH, adrenocorticotrophic hormone; CRH, corticotropin-releasing hormone; DDAVP, desmopressin acetate; iMAD, isolated micronodular adrenocortical disease; PPNAD, primary pigmented adrenocortical nodular disease.

be used postoperatively for monitoring of recurrence. For neuronal origin tumors that may secrete ACTH and/or CRH, chromogranin A (CrgA) is a useful marker.

After the establishment of the diagnosis of endogenous CS, ACTH levels should be measured to differentiate between ACTH-dependent (usually ACTH > 30 pg/mL) or ACTH-independent causes (suppressed ACTH <5 pg/mL). In ACTH-dependent CS, an MRI of the pituitary along with high-dose dexamethasone suppression test (8 mg or equivalent weight-based dose of 120 µg/kg in children) and the CRH test are used to define the source of hypercortisolemia as either in the pituitary or ectopic. If those results are inconclusive, bilateral inferior petrosal sinus sampling could assist in defining the source of hypercortisolemia.[2]

In cases of ACTH-independent CS, imaging of the adrenals is the next diagnostic step to assess the presence of a unilateral tumor or bilateral adrenal disease. Ultrasound imaging of the adrenals has not been proven to be sensitive in identifying adrenal masses beyond large ACTs and sizable carcinomas; thus, computed tomography scans primarily (sensitive for small lesions of <1 cm) or MRI (not as good for lesions <1 cm owing to motion artifacts) are the recommended imaging modalities. In the presence of bilateral adrenal disease or in cases of intermediate levels of ACTH, the standard 6-day low- and high-dose dexamethasone suppression test (Liddle test) is used to differentiate between the various causes of CS. Calculation of the level of suppression of serum cortisol levels, and urinary free cortisol and 17-hydroxy steroids can lead toward a specific cause.[2,71]

In more complicated cases, additional imaging studies, such as PET scan with [8]F-fluorodeoxyglucose, octreotide scan, or imaging studies of additional parts of the body may be indicated.[70]

MANAGEMENT OF CUSHING SYNDROME

The management of neonatal CS depends on the underlying cause of the disease. Although in the past the survival rate of neonates and infants diagnosed with CS was low (Supplemental Table 1), the advances of medicine have improved this over the last decades.

Adrenocortical carcinomas are managed with laparoscopic or open (depending on the size of the tumor and the suspicion of local invasion) complete en bloc resection of the primary tumor and the peritumoral/periadrenal retroperitoneal fat, and adjuvant chemotherapy with mitotane.[72–74] Benign adrenal tumors are usually managed with surgical resection with no need for additional treatment.

In cases of bilateral adrenal hyperplasia, patients are managed with bilateral adrenalectomy, which requires life-long GC and mineralocorticoid replacement. Unilateral adrenalectomy or bilateral partial adrenalectomy has been also suggested as an alternative option, reserving the endogenous GC production.[75] However, in these cases, regular monitoring for recurrence of CS should be undertaken. In CS associated with MAS specifically, given the possibility of spontaneous resolution of the disease, initial medical management or subtotal adrenalectomy could be attempted to preserve the adrenal function later in life.[76]

Pituitary corticotropinomas are generally managed with transsphenoidal resection with a high rate of success in specialized centers.[77,78] A transsphenoidal resection approach, however, is difficult in young infants, given the limited space in the nostrils and the lack of pneumatization of the sphenoid sinus, which starts around the age of 2 years. Thus, a transcranial approach to the pituitary is usually required. Recently, the transsphenoidal approach has been successfully used even in young infants and provides an alternative less invasive technique.[79] Given the possibility of pituitary hormone deficiencies as a result of the manipulation of the pituitary gland and their long-term effects in the developing child, referral to a center with a neurosurgeon specialized in pediatric tumors is highly recommended. In cases of persistent disease, repeat surgery may be considered, but the success rate is lower (60%) and the possibility of persistent pituitary hormone deficiencies is greater.[38,80] If hypercortisolemia persists, then radiation or medical treatment (ketoconazole, metyrapone, mitotane, mifepristone) are additional options to control the hypercortisolemia.[81]

Postoperatively, the patients require GC replacement with hydrocortisone until the recovery of the HPA is documented, which usually requires 12 to 18 months.[82] Documentation of recovery is based on a normal 8 AM serum cortisol level (>6 µg/dL) or a sufficient response of cortisol production (>18 µg/dL) after administration of cosyntropin.[83]

Despite the resolution of hypercortisolemia, patients with history of CS present with persistent features that need life long monitoring.[77] Those include persistent elevation of body mass index, several risk factors for the metabolic syndrome (hypertension, hyperlipidemia, and impaired glucose tolerance), bone manifestations, and cognitive and psychological problems.[77]

SUMMARY

Neonatal CS is a rare condition in the neonate and infantile period. It is usually caused by an adrenal disease, often ACT. Genetic causes explain a large portion of the patients, and the clinical presentation of the patient should guide appropriate genetic testing, which is important for the prognosis and follow-up evaluation. The diagnostic evaluation of CS should follow the recommended steps to distinguish ACTH-dependent from ACTH-independent etiologies, identify early cancer, and guide the appropriate management of the patient. Although surgical management of the source of hypercortisolemia may result in cure, long-term manifestations of CS may persist and require regular monitoring.

Best Practices

What is the current practice?

- CS is suspected on the basis of the patient's clinical presentation (see **Table 2**).

- Confirmation of hypercortisolemia requires at least 2 abnormal results in the screening tests:
  1. Abnormal circadian rhythm of cortisol secretion (may not be definitive at age of <1 year);
  2. Elevated urine free cortisol levels; and
  3. Lack of suppression of cortisol production after dexamethasone administration.

- After confirmation of hypercortisolemia, further evaluation of the source is suggested according to the diagnostic algorithm in **Fig. 3**.

What changes in current practice are likely to improve outcomes?

- Prompt genetic testing of the patients.

- Surgical approaches that involve adrenal sparing for patients with bilateral adrenal disease.

Is there a clinical algorithm?

See **Fig. 3** for the established diagnostic algorithm of patients with suspected CS.

Summary Statement

Neonatal CS is usually caused by exogenous administration of GCs and rarely by endogenous hypercortisolemia. Adrenal CS is the most common cause of endogenous CS in neonates and infants, and ACTs represent the majority of cases. Many of the ACTs develop in the context of a *TP53* gene mutation, which causes Li-Fraumeni syndrome. More rarely, neonatal CS presents as part of other syndromes such as MAS or BWS. The management of the patients usually includes resection of the primary tumor with or without additional medical treatment, but various manifestations may persist after resolution of hypercortisolemia.

SUPPLEMENTARY DATA

Supplementary data related to this article can be found online at https://doi.org/10.1016/j.clp.2017.10.002.

REFERENCES

1. Lindholm J. Cushing's syndrome: historical aspects. Pituitary 2000;3(2):97–104.
2. Stratakis CA. Diagnosis and clinical genetics of Cushing syndrome in pediatrics. Endocrinol Metab Clin North America 2016;45(2):311–28.
3. Hench P. Effects of cortisone in the rheumatic diseases. Lancet 1950;2(6634): 483–4.
4. Schappert SM, Rechtsteiner EA. Ambulatory medical care utilization estimates for 2006. Natl Health Stat Report 2008;(8):1–29.
5. Stratakis CA. Cushing syndrome in pediatrics. Endocrinol Metab Clin North Am 2012;41(4):793–803.
6. Villee DB. Development of endocrine function in the human placenta and fetus (first of two parts). N Engl J Med 1969;281(9):473–84.
7. Ross IL, Louw GJ. Embryological and molecular development of the adrenal glands. Clin Anat 2015;28(2):235–42.
8. Ferraz-de-Souza B, Achermann JC. Disorders of adrenal development. Endocr Dev 2008;13:19–32.
9. Buster JE. Fetal adrenal cortex. Clin Obstet Gynecol 1980;23(3):803–24.
10. Seron-Ferre M, Jaffe RB. The fetal adrenal gland. Annu Rev Physiol 1981;43: 141–62.
11. Melmed S, Polonsky K, Larsen PR, et al. Endocrinology of fetal development. Chapter 22. 12th edition. Williams Textbook of Endocrinology; 2011. p. 833–67.
12. Fisher DA. The unique endocrine milieu of the fetus. J Clin Invest 1986;78(3): 603–11.
13. Mesiano S, Jaffe RB. Developmental and functional biology of the primate fetal adrenal cortex. Endocr Rev 1997;18(3):378–403.
14. Liggins GC. Adrenocortical-related maturational events in the fetus. Am J Obstet Gynecol 1976;126(7):931–41.
15. Dotzler SA, Digeronimo RJ, Yoder BA, et al. Distribution of corticotropin releasing hormone in the fetus, newborn, juvenile, and adult baboon. Pediatr Res 2004; 55(1):120–5.
16. Goland RS, Wardlaw SL, Blum M, et al. Biologically active corticotropin-releasing hormone in maternal and fetal plasma during pregnancy. Am J Obstet Gynecol 1988;159(4):884–90.
17. Tsigos C, Chrousos GP. Differential diagnosis and management of Cushing's syndrome. Annu Rev Med 1996;47:443–61.
18. Orth DN. Cushing's syndrome. N Engl J Med 1995;332(12):791–803.
19. Lim CT, Grossman A, Khoo B. Normal physiology of ACTH and GH release in the hypothalamus and anterior pituitary in man. In: De Groot LJ, Chrousos G, Dungan K, et al, editors. Endotext [Internet]. South Dartmouth (MA): MDText.com, Inc; 2000. Available from: https://www.ncbi.nlm.nih.gov/books/NBK279116/. Accessed November 22, 2017.
20. Buckley TM, Schatzberg AF. On the interactions of the hypothalamic-pituitary-adrenal (HPA) axis and sleep: normal HPA axis activity and circadian rhythm, exemplary sleep disorders. J Clin Endocrinol Metab 2005;90(5):3106–14.
21. Seckl JR. Prenatal glucocorticoids and long-term programming. Eur J Endocrinol 2004;151(Suppl 3):U49–62.

22. Baud O, Sola A. Corticosteroids in perinatal medicine: how to improve outcomes without affecting the developing brain? Semin Fetal Neonatal Med 2007;12(4): 273–9.

23. Rajadurai VS, Tan KH. The use and abuse of steroids in perinatal medicine. Ann Acad Med Singapore 2003;32(3):324–34.

24. Onland W, De Jaegere AP, Offringa M, et al. Systemic corticosteroid regimens for prevention of bronchopulmonary dysplasia in preterm infants. Cochrane Database Syst Rev 2017;(1):CD010941.

25. Ermis B, Ors R, Tastekin A, et al. Cushing's syndrome secondary to topical corticosteroids abuse. Clin Endocrinol (Oxf) 2003;58(6):795–6.

26. Ribeiro RC, Pinto EM, Zambetti GP, et al. The International Pediatric Adrenocortical Tumor Registry initiative: contributions to clinical, biological, and treatment advances in pediatric adrenocortical tumors. Mol Cell Endocrinol 2012;351(1): 37–43.

27. Sandrini R, Ribeiro RC, DeLacerda L. Childhood adrenocortical tumors. J Clin Endocrinol Metab 1997;82(7):2027–31.

28. Chen QL, Su Z, Li YH, et al. Clinical characteristics of adrenocortical tumors in children. J Pediatr Endocrinol Metab 2011;24(7–8):535–41.

29. Stratakis CA, Boikos SA. Genetics of adrenal tumors associated with Cushing's syndrome: a new classification for bilateral adrenocortical hyperplasias. Nat Clin Pract Endocrinol Metab 2007;3(11):748–57.

30. Stratakis CA. Cushing syndrome caused by adrenocortical tumors and hyperplasias (corticotropin- independent Cushing syndrome). Endocr Dev 2008;13: 117–32.

31. Gkourogianni A, Sinaii N, Jackson SH, et al. Pediatric Cushing disease: disparities in disease severity and outcomes in the Hispanic and African-American populations. Pediatr Res 2017. https://doi.org/10.1038/pr.2017.58.

32. Libuit LG, Karageorgiadis AS, Sinaii N, et al. A gender-dependent analysis of Cushing's disease in childhood: pre- and postoperative follow-up. Clin Endocrinol (Oxf) 2015;83(1):72–7.

33. Lodish M, Stratakis CA. A genetic and molecular update on adrenocortical causes of Cushing syndrome. Nat Rev Endocrinol 2016;12(5):255–62.

34. de Kock L, Sabbaghian N, Plourde F, et al. Pituitary blastoma: a pathognomonic feature of germ-line DICER1 mutations. Acta Neuropathol 2014;128(1):111–22.

35. Scheithauer BW, Horvath E, Abel TW, et al. Pituitary blastoma: a unique embryonal tumor. Pituitary 2012;15(3):365–73.

36. Karageorgiadis AS, Papadakis GZ, Biro J, et al. Ectopic adrenocorticotropic hormone and corticotropin-releasing hormone co-secreting tumors in children and adolescents causing Cushing syndrome: a diagnostic dilemma and how to solve it. J Clin Endocrinol Metab 2015;100(1):141–8.

37. Espinasse-Holder M, Defachelles AS, Weill J, et al. Paraneoplastic Cushing syndrome due to adrenal neuroblastoma. Med Pediatr Oncol 2000;34(3):231–3.

38. Lodish M. Cushing's syndrome in childhood: update on genetics, treatment, and outcomes. Curr Opin Endocrinol Diabetes Obes 2015;22(1):48–54.

39. Gonzalez KD, Noltner KA, Buzin CH, et al. Beyond Li Fraumeni syndrome: clinical characteristics of families with p53 germline mutations. J Clin Oncol 2009;27(8): 1250–6.

40. Ribeiro RC, Sandrini F, Figueiredo B, et al. An inherited p53 mutation that contributes in a tissue-specific manner to pediatric adrenal cortical carcinoma. Proc Natl Acad Sci U S A 2001;98(16):9330–5.

41. Latronico AC, Pinto EM, Domenice S, et al. An inherited mutation outside the highly conserved DNA-binding domain of the p53 tumor suppressor protein in children and adults with sporadic adrenocortical tumors. J Clin Endocrinol Metab 2001;86(10):4970–3.
42. Li FP, Fraumeni JF Jr, Mulvihill JJ, et al. A cancer family syndrome in twenty-four kindreds. Cancer Res 1988;48(18):5358–62.
43. Mai PL, Best AF, Peters JA, et al. Risks of first and subsequent cancers among TP53 mutation carriers in the National Cancer Institute Li-Fraumeni syndrome cohort. Cancer 2016;122(23):3673–81.
44. Dumitrescu CE, Collins MT. McCune-Albright syndrome. Orphanet J Rare Dis 2008;3:12.
45. Brown RJ, Kelly MH, Collins MT. Cushing syndrome in the McCune-Albright syndrome. J Clin Endocrinol Metab 2010;95(4):1508–15.
46. Carney JA, Young WF, Stratakis CA. Primary bimorphic adrenocortical disease: cause of hypercortisolism in McCune-Albright syndrome. Am J Surg Pathol 2011;35(9):1311–26.
47. Kirschner LS, Carney JA, Pack SD, et al. Mutations of the gene encoding the protein kinase A type I-alpha regulatory subunit in patients with the Carney complex. Nat Genet 2000;26(1):89–92.
48. Stratakis CA. Carney complex: a familial lentiginosis predisposing to a variety of tumors. Rev Endocr Metab Disord 2016;17(3):367–71.
49. Gicquel C, Bertagna X, Schneid H, et al. Rearrangements at the 11p15 locus and overexpression of insulin-like growth factor-II gene in sporadic adrenocortical tumors. J Clin Endocrinol Metab 1994;78(6):1444–53.
50. Shuman C, Beckwith JB, Weksberg R. Beckwith-Wiedemann syndrome. In: Pagon RA, Adam MP, Ardinger HH, et al, editors. GeneReviews(R). Seattle (WA): 1993.
51. MacFarland SP, Mostoufi-Moab S, Zelley K, et al. Management of adrenal masses in patients with Beckwith-Wiedemann syndrome. Pediatr Blood Cancer 2017; 64(8). https://doi.org/10.1002/pbc.26432.
52. Carney JA, Ho J, Kitsuda K, et al. Massive neonatal adrenal enlargement due to cytomegaly, persistence of the transient cortex, and hyperplasia of the permanent cortex: findings in Cushing syndrome associated with hemihypertrophy. Am J Surg Pathol 2012;36(10):1452–63.
53. Brioude F, Nicolas C, Marey I, et al. Hypercortisolism due to a pituitary adenoma associated with Beckwith-Wiedemann syndrome. Horm Res Paediatr 2016;86(3): 206–11.
54. Ribeiro RC, Pinto EM, Zambetti GP. Familial predisposition to adrenocortical tumors: clinical and biological features and management strategies. Best Pract Res Clin Endocrinol Metab 2010;24(3):477–90.
55. Almeida MQ, Latronico AC. The molecular pathogenesis of childhood adrenocortical tumors. Horm Metab Res 2007;39(6):461–6.
56. Stratakis CA, Tichomirowa MA, Boikos S, et al. The role of germline AIP, MEN1, PRKAR1A, CDKN1B and CDKN2C mutations in causing pituitary adenomas in a large cohort of children, adolescents, and patients with genetic syndromes. Clin Genet 2010;78(5):457–63.
57. Reincke M, Sbiera S, Hayakawa A, et al. Mutations in the deubiquitinase gene USP8 cause Cushing's disease. Nat Genet 2015;47(1):31–8.
58. Faucz FR, Tirosh A, Tatsi C, et al. Somatic USP8 gene mutations are a common cause of pediatric Cushing disease. J Clin Endocrinol Metab 2017. https://doi.org/10.1210/jc.2017-00161.

59. Foulkes WD, Priest JR, Duchaine TF. DICER1: mutations, microRNAs and mechanisms. Nat Rev Cancer 2014;14(10):662–72.

60. Magiakou MA, Mastorakos G, Oldfield EH, et al. Cushing's syndrome in children and adolescents. Presentation, diagnosis, and therapy. N Engl J Med 1994; 331(10):629–36.

61. Stratakis CA, Mastorakos G, Mitsiades NS, et al. Skin manifestations of Cushing disease in children and adolescents before and after the resolution of hypercortisolemia. Pediatr Dermatol 1998;15(4):253–8.

62. Tack LJ, Tatsi C, Stratakis CA, et al. Effects of glucocorticoids on bone: what we can learn from pediatric endogenous Cushing's syndrome. Horm Metab Res 2016;48(11):764–70.

63. Magiakou MA, Mastorakos G, Chrousos GP. Final stature in patients with endogenous Cushing's syndrome. J Clin Endocrinol Metab 1994;79(4):1082–5.

64. Oppong E, Cato AC. Effects of glucocorticoids in the immune system. Adv Exp Med Biol 2015;872:217–33.

65. Gkourogianni A, Lodish MB, Zilbermint M, et al. Death in pediatric Cushing syndrome is uncommon but still occurs. Eur J Pediatr 2015;174(4):501–7.

66. Scaroni C, Zilio M, Foti M, et al. Glucose metabolism abnormalities in Cushing syndrome: from molecular basis to clinical management. Endocr Rev 2017; 38(3):189–219.

67. Lodish MB, Sinaii N, Patronas N, et al. Blood pressure in pediatric patients with Cushing syndrome. J Clin Endocrinol Metab 2009;94(6):2002–8.

68. Nguyen JH, Lodish MB, Patronas NJ, et al. Extensive and largely reversible ischemic cerebral infarctions in a prepubertal child with hypertension and Cushing disease. J Clin Endocrinol Metab 2009;94(1):1–2.

69. Bartz SK, Karaviti LP, Brandt ML, et al. Residual manifestations of hypercortisolemia following surgical treatment in a patient with Cushing syndrome. Int J Pediatr Endocrinol 2015;2015(1):19.

70. Lacroix A, Feelders RA, Stratakis CA, et al. Cushing's syndrome. Lancet 2015; 386(9996):913–27.

71. Stratakis CA, Sarlis N, Kirschner LS, et al. Paradoxical response to dexamethasone in the diagnosis of primary pigmented nodular adrenocortical disease. Ann Intern Med 1999;131(8):585–91.

72. Berruti A, Baudin E, Gelderblom H, et al. Adrenal cancer: ESMO clinical practice guidelines for diagnosis, treatment and follow-up. Ann Oncol 2012;23(Suppl 7): vii131–8.

73. Gaujoux S, Mihai R, Joint Working Group of ESES and ENSAT. European Society of Endocrine Surgeons (ESES) and European Network for the Study of Adrenal Tumours (ENSAT) recommendations for the surgical management of adrenocortical carcinoma. Br J Surg 2017;104(4):358–76.

74. Berruti A, Grisanti S, Pulzer A, et al. Long-term outcomes of adjuvant mitotane therapy in patients with radically resected adrenocortical carcinoma. J Clin Endocrinol Metab 2017;102(4):1358–65.

75. Lowery AJ, Seeliger B, Alesina PF, et al. Posterior retroperitoneoscopic adrenal surgery for clinical and subclinical Cushing's syndrome in patients with bilateral adrenal disease. Langenbecks Arch Surg 2017. https://doi.org/10.1007/s00423-017-1569-6.

76. Itonaga T, Goto H, Toujigamori M, et al. Three-quarters adrenalectomy for infantile-onset Cushing syndrome due to bilateral adrenal hyperplasia in McCune-Albright syndrome. Horm Res Paediatr 2017. https://doi.org/10.1159/000473878.

77. Keil MF. Quality of life and other outcomes in children treated for Cushing syndrome. J Clin Endocrinol Metab 2013;98(7):2667–78.
78. Chandler WF, Barkan AL, Hollon T, et al. Outcome of transsphenoidal surgery for Cushing disease: a single-center experience over 32 years. Neurosurgery 2016; 78(2):216–23.
79. Zaben M, Zafar M, Bukhari S, et al. Endoscopic transsphenoidal approach for resection of malignant pituitary blastoma in an 18-month-old infant: a technical note. Neurosurgery 2014;10(Suppl 4):649–53.
80. Lonser RR, Wind JJ, Nieman LK, et al. Outcome of surgical treatment of 200 children with Cushing's disease. J Clin Endocrinol Metab 2013;98(3):892–901.
81. Feelders RA, Hofland LJ. Medical treatment of Cushing's disease. J Clin Endocrinol Metab 2013;98(2):425–38.
82. Lodish M, Dunn SV, Sinaii N, et al. Recovery of the hypothalamic-pituitary-adrenal axis in children and adolescents after surgical cure of Cushing's disease. J Clin Endocrinol Metab 2012;97(5):1483–91.
83. Bornstein SR, Allolio B, Arlt W, et al. Diagnosis and treatment of primary adrenal insufficiency: an Endocrine Society clinical practice guideline. J Clin Endocrinol Metab 2016;101(2):364–89.

Turner Syndrome
Diagnostic and Management Considerations for Perinatal Clinicians

Jacob M. Redel, MD, Philippe F. Backeljauw, MD*

KEYWORDS

- Turner syndrome • Monosomy X • Perinatology • Karyotype • Counseling

KEY POINTS

- Clinical features of Turner Syndrome require immediate genetic testing.
- The diagnosis of Turner Syndrome is made postnatally via 30 cell karyotype.
- Screening for cardiac and renal abnormalities is necessary soon after diagnosis.
- Counseling families after diagnosis of Turner Syndrome is challenging, but is an essential part of perinatal care for these patients.

INTRODUCTION

Turner syndrome (TS) is a common genetic condition resulting from absence of all or part of the second sex chromosome.[1,2] Patients with TS commonly exhibit cardiovascular, endocrine, renal, reproductive, autoimmune, hearing, vision, and/or psychosocial abnormalities, among other conditions.[1] Although there is a wide spectrum of disease severity, essentially all individuals require ongoing involvement with multiple subspecialists throughout their lifetimes. Early recognition and diagnosis is valuable in helping to screen for complications, establish specialty care, and provide optimal counseling for families.

The prevalence of TS is reported to be approximately 1 in 2000 to 1 in 2500 live female births.[2,3] Further, aneuploidy is a common cause of spontaneous abortion, so the incidence among all conceptions is much higher.[4] Perinatal physicians are highly likely to encounter these patients in their practice. Understanding how to recognize, diagnose, and manage individuals with TS early in life and how to appropriately counsel their families, is essential in providing optimal care to these patients.

Disclosure Statement: The authors have no relevant disclosures to report.
Division of Endocrinology, Cincinnati Children's Hospital Medical Center, The University of Cincinnati College of Medicine, 3333 Burnet Avenue, Cincinnati, OH 45229, USA
* Corresponding author. 3333 Burnet Avenue, MLC 7012, Cincinnati, OH 45229.
E-mail address: philippe.backeljauw@cchmc.org

Clin Perinatol 45 (2018) 119–128
https://doi.org/10.1016/j.clp.2017.11.003
perinatology.theclinics.com

DIAGNOSIS
Diagnostic Criteria

Early diagnosis of TS provides the best opportunity for recognition and intervention of potential abnormalities. Delayed diagnosis can significantly impact the health-related quality of life for these patients.[1] According to the clinical practice guidelines recently published in the *European Journal of Endocrinology*, diagnosis of TS is made in phenotypic girls who have at least 1 X chromosome, complete or partial absence of the second sex chromosome, and at least 1 characteristic clinical manifestation.[1] Exceptions to these criteria include (1) individuals with a male phenotype or (2) girls with a second X chromosome having a deletion distal to Xq24.[1] Girls with such a deletion generally have premature ovarian failure but do not exhibit other clinical features of TS, neither in the neonatal period nor later in life. Clinical features that indicate TS (**Table 1**) should prompt cytogenetic testing (karyotype analysis) in the neonatal period. When testing girls with these characteristic features, a positive result with 5% or greater mosaicism meets the genetic criteria for diagnosis.[1]

Prenatal Diagnosis

The diagnosis of TS is commonly made postnatally after characteristic features are recognized. However, some fetuses are screened prenatally because of problems during gestation or during high-risk pregnancies. In these cases, the preliminary diagnosis is usually made via karyotype analysis after chorionic villus sampling or amniocentesis. Additionally, ultrasonography can suggest a diagnosis of TS in utero, as findings of increased nuchal translucency, cystic hygroma, aortic/left-sided heart defects, brachycephaly, renal dysplasia (including horseshoe kidney), polyhydramnios, and oligohydramnios are all features that make the diagnosis of TS more likely. A mild degree of smallness for gestational age can be also be a sign of TS, as infants with TS are born with lower weights/lengths on average than other infants.[5] Regardless of the prenatal findings, karyotype should always be performed postnatally to confirm the diagnosis.

Even in the absence of significant risk factors, prenatal screening tests are more commonly being offered during pregnancy. Maternal serum triple and quadruple screens may detect TS (among other conditions) by measuring concentrations of α-fetoprotein, human chorionic gonadotropin, inhibin A, and estriol.

Table 1
Clinical features of Turner Syndrome in the neonatal period that should prompt strong consideration for postnatal karyotyping

System Affected	Clinical Manifestation
General	Failure to thrive, growth failure
Lymphatic	Cystic hygroma, hydrops, lymphedema of extremities (hands/feet)
Cardiovascular	Left-sided heart defects, especially aortic arch abnormalities and bicuspid aortic valve
Mouth	Micrognathia, high-arched palate
Head and face	Epicanthal folds, ptosis, strabismus, external ear deformities, low set ears
Chest	Shield chest, wide-spaced nipples
Neck	Neck webbing, short neck, low posterior hairline
Renal	Horseshoe kidney, collecting duct abnormality, ectopic kidney
Extremities	Edema, Madelung deformity, nail dysplasia/hypoplasia

Additionally, noninvasive prenatal screening using cell-free DNA, is now being offered to pregnant women to detect aneuploidy. However, as with amniocentesis and chorionic villus sampling, postnatal karyotype analysis should always be performed to confirm the diagnosis. Cell-free DNA is highly accurate for detection of trisomy, with both sensitivity and specificity reported at greater than 99%.[6] However, the sensitivity for detecting monosomy is lower, at 95.8%.[6]

Postnatal Diagnosis

A postnatal karyotype should be performed on all patients with positive prenatal screening findings or clinical examination features concerning for TS.[1] The diagnosis cannot be made definitively without this testing. The American College of Medical Genetics recommends a 30-cell analysis be performed for routine karyotype because of the high rate of mosaicism in TS.[7] Classically, a patient with TS has a complete absence of the second sex chromosome, resulting in a karyotype of 45,X. However, there are several variations from this classical karyotype also diagnostic for TS. The most common karyotypes that define a diagnosis of TS are outlined in **Table 2**. Of note, most patients with TS have some degree of mosaicism. Generally, the clinical findings in patients with mosaicism are milder than in patients who have the 45,X genotype present in all cells. Different tissues also may have different degrees of mosaicism. Lack of mosaicism in a peripheral blood sample does not necessarily mean the patient has no mosaicism in other tissues. Thus, it is possible, albeit uncommon, for a patient with TS to have a normal karyotype on the peripheral blood sample. In cases of high clinical suspicion for TS after a normal

Table 2
Most common karyotypes found in Turner Syndrome

Karyotype	Description	Prevalence (% of Live Births)
45,X	Complete absence of second sex chromosome	40–50
45,X/46,XX	TS mosaicism with normal karyotype	15–25
45,X/46,XY (Y chromosomal mosaicism)	Presence of Y chromosome material in some cells. If all cells contain Y chromosome material, the diagnosis is not consistent with TS	10–12
Isochrome Xq (i(X)q); Isodicentric Xp (idic(Xp))	Presence of 2 copies of the long arm (q) of the X chromosome, with complete or near-complete lack of the short arm (p) of X; Absence or near-absence of Xq	10
45,X/47,XXX; 45,X/46, XX/47,XXX	XXX mosaicism	3
Ring chromosome X (rX)	A ring formed if parts of both the long and short arm of the X chromosome are missing	—
Xp deletion (del(X)p)	Partial or complete deletion of the short arm (p) of X	—
Xq deletion (del(X)q)	Partial or complete deletion of the long arm (q) of X (not TS if Xq24 or distal)	—

Adapted from Gravholt CH, Andersen NH, Conway GS, et al. Clinical practice guidelines for the care of girls and women with Turner syndrome: proceedings from the 2016 Cincinnati International Turner Syndrome Meeting. Eur J Endocrinol 2017;177(3):G9; with permission.

46,XX karyotype from a blood sample, further cytogenetic analysis by skin biopsy or buccal smear may be considered.[7]

It is additionally important to recognize whether the karyotype result shows presence of any Y chromosome material or whether the patient has clinical findings of virilization. Presence of the Y chromosome is associated with a significantly elevated risk for gonadoblastoma.[8] Even if the karyotype does not identify Y chromosome mosaicism, clinical virilization (clitoromegaly or sexual ambiguity) in a patient with TS is highly suggestive for presence of Y chromosome material. In those situations, further testing must be performed. Fluorescence in situ hybridization for Y chromosome is the preferred method of detecting Y chromosome material.[7] No individual gene (such as SRY) has yet been found to be associated with gonadoblastoma formation risk, so specific gene testing is not currently recommended.[1] If Y chromosome material is present, prophylactic gonadectomy is recommended early in life.[1,8]

PERINATAL EVALUATION

Patients with TS require a multidisciplinary evaluation by several pediatric subspecialists. Much of this evaluation can be performed in the outpatient setting. However, testing for cardiac and renal anomalies should be performed in the perinatal period. These evaluations should always be conducted as soon as possible after initial diagnosis.

Cardiovascular Evaluation

Cardiac anomalies are common in girls with TS, found in approximately 50% of this population.[1] All infants with TS should have electrocardiography and echocardiogram performed in conjunction with evaluation by a cardiologist. Early identification of congenital heart defects is essential, as this is a major source of morbidity and mortality in patients with TS.[9,10] A bicuspid aortic valve and aorta abnormalities (coarctation, dilation, and elongation of the transverse aorta) are the most common defects found in TS (**Fig. 1**). In addition, several other defects are also more commonly found in this population. Some of these include ventricular septal defects, atrial septal defects, systemic and pulmonary venous abnormalities, and coronary artery abnormalities.

Of note, the phenotype of a webbed neck should alert the clinician to a higher risk of congenital heart disease. Neck webbing is found to be strongly associated with a higher risk for both bicuspid aortic valve and coarctation of the aorta, independent of postnatal karyotype.[11] Although the exact mechanism for this association is not known, it is hypothesized that altered lymphatic pressure and flow may disrupt normal left-sided cardiac development.[9,11,12]

In addition to structural defects, electric conduction abnormalities have been reported in girls with TS.[13] These include prolonged QT interval, T wave changes, and atrioventricular conduction acceleration. If conduction abnormalities are identified, medications that could exacerbate them (such as QT-prolonging medications in patients with prolonged QTc), should be avoided when possible.[13,14]

Renal Evaluation

TS is associated with congenital anomalies of the genitourinary system. All infants with TS should undergo renal ultrasound scan at the time of diagnosis. Early diagnosis of these renal anomalies prompts intervention for any problems that could impair function of the genitourinary system or could exacerbate sequelae

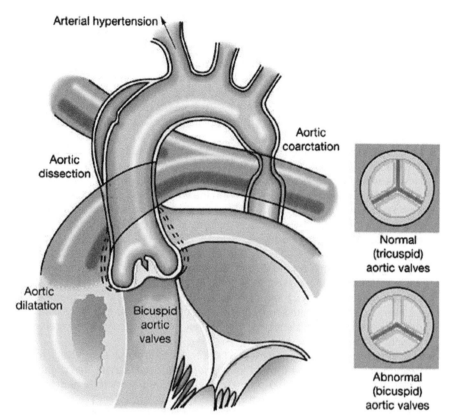

Fig. 1. Common cardiovascular anomalies in TS. (*Reprinted by permission from* Macmillan Publishers Ltd: Nat Clin Pract Endocrinol Metab. Gravholt CH. Clinical practice in Turner syndrome. Nat Clin Pract Endocrinol Metabol 2005 Nov;1(1):41–52. Copyright 2005.)

related to cardiac defects. The most common renal anomalies found in TS are abnormalities of the collecting system (such as malformation or duplication), horseshoe kidney, or positional abnormalities of the kidneys. Many of these nonobstructive anatomic anomalies do not translate into functional renal problems and in the absence of urinary tract infections may only require observation in the long term.

Other Inpatient Evaluations to Consider

- Poor weight gain. Although many TS individuals have normal birth weight, infants with TS are generally smaller at birth,[5] and have a higher risk for mild intrauterine growth retardation and poor weight gain early in life. Poor feeding habits, which may be related to a palate anatomy anomaly (a narrow palate), can result in undernutrition, preventing adequate weight gain in infancy. Thus, it is not uncommon for these infants to have failure to thrive. Close monitoring of oral intake and weight by a perinatal physician or dietician is important in supporting optimal weight gain early in life.
- Growth and skeleton. Girls with TS are at a higher risk of poor growth and abnormalities of the skeleton,[1,15,16] largely attributed to haploinsufficiency of the short

stature homeobox on the X chromosome (SHOX) gene.[1,15] This gene is an important mediator of normal growth. Loss of the SHOX gene region (Xp22.33) has been associated with shortened forearm, shortened lower leg, cubitus valgus, Madelung deformity, and high-arched narrow palate.[17] Other skeletal abnormalities associated with TS include retrognathia, sternum abnormalities, shortened fourth and/or fifth metacarpals or metatarsals, kyphoscoliosis, genu valgum, and foot abnormalities.[1,15] Additionally, TS patients may be at increased risk of hip dysplasia relative to the general population, thus a thorough clinical hip examination is recommended early in life.[1]

- Lymphedema. Lymphedema is a common finding in infants with TS. Presence of lymphedema in an infant girl should immediately raise suspicion for TS. Central lymphedema in a TS fetus with hydrops is found to be strongly associated with cardiac defects, as described above.[11] In the fetus and in infants, central lymphedema can manifest as a cystic hygroma, a webbed neck, a low posterior hairline, and rotated pinnae.[1] These features may result from disruption of flow between the jugular lymphatics and jugular vein.[11,12] Peripheral lymphedema, although not specifically associated with cardiac anomalies, can result in substantial swelling in the hands and feet. It is recommended that, if there are significant adverse effects from the edema on the skin or fingernails/toenails (nail hypoplasia, nail hyperconvexity), the patient should be treated by an edema therapist.[1] Diuretics are not indicated to treat the peripheral lymphedema in TS; they can cause dehydration and electrolyte disturbances and have not demonstrated significant benefit for the edema.[2]

- Hearing. Girls with TS are at increased risk for hearing problems.[18] Thus, routine hearing screening, as performed in all infants, is necessary in this population. Failed hearing screen should be taken seriously, with audiology and otolaryngology referral soon after these findings.

- Gonadal failure. Primary hypogonadism is found in a large majority of girls with TS and causes delayed puberty, infertility, and poor bone density later in life.[19] Although ovarian failure does not result in significant problems until the pubertal age range, one may wish to screen for primary hypogonadism to assist with prognosis and counseling. Testing for primary hypogonadism can best be performed at 2 to 3 months of age, as this period captures the normally observed physiologic increase in gonadotropin concentrations after the first 4 to 6 weeks of life. Measurement of luteinizing hormone, follicle-stimulating hormone, estradiol, and anti-Müllerian hormone may be performed during this time if the clinician and family wish to evaluate gonadal function.[20,21] Abnormal values can be helpful in counseling the family about the high likelihood of early ovarian failure and infertility. On the contrary, normal laboratory results during infancy should be reviewed with caution, as they do not exclude hypogonadism later in life. The above laboratory values will usually need to be repeated starting at 11 years of age to determine whether to initiate estrogen replacement therapy at that time.[1] Fertility counseling may be initiated during late childhood, as oocyte cryopreservation is an option for girls who retain ovarian function at 12 years of age.[1]

COUNSELING AND LONG-TERM HEALTH OUTCOMES

Initial counseling of families who have a child with TS can be challenging. The goal for the first discussion between a perinatal clinician and family should be to promptly disclose the diagnosis and accurately, yet succinctly, convey essential comorbidity information about TS. The challenges encountered in the process of discussing this diagnosis have resulted in some families feeling as if they were not adequately informed—or worse—that the diagnosis was withheld from them for some time.[22] Therefore, shortly after initial disclosure of the diagnosis, families should be counseled again, so that they understand what having TS means for the child and the family. This discussion should include (1) an explanation of the underlying genetics at a level appropriate for the family's medical literacy, (2) the reason for perinatal evaluations and testing (including prompt cardiac and renal imaging), (3) the eventual need to screen for a variety of other problems, and (4) the high likelihood of long-term health care needs, especially with respect to growth delay and ovarian failure. Over time, less common or less severe clinical manifestations should also be introduced. For example, the propensity for anxiety and attention deficit problems in girls with TS should be discussed eventually but does not need to be a part of the initial counseling.

In-depth discussion should preferably be conducted by a specialist with extensive experience in treating patients with TS. Pediatric endocrinologists have the most expertise, as they are involved in managing multiple aspects of the long-term care of TS (including growth failure, ovarian failure, bone health, and screening for comorbidities such as thyroid autoimmune disease). Additionally, a geneticist or genetic counselor can provide assistance to clinicians when thorough genetic counseling about TS is needed. Online resources and information about advocacy groups can be beneficial to families of girls with TS. For patients in the United States, we recommend providing information for the TS Society of the United States (www.turnersyndrome.org) or the TS Foundation (www.turnersyndromefoundation.org).

SUMMARY

The perinatal period is a crucial time for identifying patients with TS. Early recognition, although not always easy to achieve, is instrumental in optimizing care for these patients. Although there are many subtle aspects of comprehensive TS management, the perinatal clinician's primary role is to identify clinical features and, when indicated, promptly do genetic testing. If not identified early in life, TS is often not diagnosed until growth failure or pubertal delay occur in late childhood or the teenage years, respectively.[23] Establishing a diagnosis early in life can make a profound difference for the clinical outcomes and quality of life for girls with TS.[1]

Karyotype analysis should be performed for any infant who has prenatal screening results indicating TS or postnatal clinical features suspicious for TS. After the diagnosis is confirmed genetically, it is essential that the perinatal physician evaluate the TS infant for cardiac anomalies (using echocardiogram and electrocardiogram) and for renal abnormalities (using renal ultrasound scan). Each newly diagnosed TS infant should be seen by a cardiologist, given the intricacies of the neonatal cardiac evaluation and blood pressure measurement interpretation. If the renal ultrasonography does not show any abnormalities with the kidney or urinary collecting system, a nephrology referral is not necessary. Early involvement with a pediatric endocrinologist is helpful for initiating a complete workup including timed evaluation of gonadal function, establishing long-term care, and facilitating appropriate counseling.

Perinatal counseling in a family not previously aware of the diagnosis should focus on defining TS, explaining the necessity for perinatal screening tests, and conveying the chronicity of the condition. The initial counseling, in most cases, should include discussion about expectations for growth failure and ovarian dysfunction to occur later in life. Online information and advocacy organization information should be provided in the initial discussion as well. Introduction of resources is important for families to have reliable resources to review at their own pace. If available, in-depth counseling by a physician with expertise in TS can be extremely valuable.

Perinatal care providers are likely to encounter multiple infants with TS during their career. These clinicians have a unique opportunity to diagnose—and intervene—very early in a TS girl's life. In addition, after making the diagnosis, these providers are likely to provide the initial counseling for families. Understanding the general principles outlined above regarding diagnosis, screening, and family counseling can help to dramatically improve the long-term outcomes for girls with TS.

Best Practices

What is the current practice?

- Newborns with features suggestive of TS should undergo cytogenetic analysis (karyotype).
- Newborns with a prenatal diagnosis of TS should undergo postnatal karyotyping.
- After diagnosis, consultation/referral is made to endocrinology and cardiology.
- Counseling of families is usually performed in the newborn unit, although the depth of discussion can vary significantly.

Best Practice Recommendations:

- Thirty-cell karyotype analysis should always be performed to make the diagnosis.
- Immediately after diagnosis, all infants should have an evaluation by a cardiologist and undergo a renal ultrasound scan.
- A pediatric endocrinologist, if available, should be consulted to assist with the workup and counseling after the initial diagnosis. Counseling should be performed at the time of diagnosis.
- Evaluation for poor weight gain, growth failure, skeletal abnormalities, lymphedema, hearing impairment, and gonadal failure should all be part of the evaluation for infants with TS.

What changes in current practice are likely to improve outcomes?

- Earlier recognition of more subtle clinical features of TS would facilitate earlier diagnosis.
- Immediate inpatient consultation by a cardiologist and a renal ultrasound scan should be performed in all TS infants so that high-risk conditions may be quickly addressed.
- Endocrinology consultation should ideally occur before discharge to assist with initial workup, counseling, and coordination of care.
- Counseling should focus on the basic genetics of the condition, the reasons for the initial workup, and the high likelihood for long-term health care needs.

Summary Statement:

TS is a relatively common genetic condition, and the perinatal period is an important opportunity for clinicians to make the diagnosis of TS. An early diagnosis can help to identify cardiovascular or genitourinary anomalies, which may otherwise result in significant morbidity/ mortality. Additionally, an early diagnosis of TS allows for comprehensive screening, care coordination, and counseling of families. Understanding the principles related to recognition, diagnosis, screening, and counseling in the perinatal period can dramatically improve outcomes and quality of life for children with TS.

REFERENCES

1. Gravholt CH, Andersen NH, Conway GS, et al. Clinical practice guidelines for the care of girls and women with Turner syndrome: proceedings from the 2016 Cincinnati International Turner Syndrome Meeting. Eur J Endocrinol 2017;177(3): G1–70.
2. Bondy CA, Turner Syndrome Study Group. Care of girls and women with turner syndrome: a guideline of the Turner syndrome study group. J Clin Endocrinol Metab 2007;92(1):10–25.
3. Nielsen J, Wohlert M. Chromosome abnormalities found among 34,910 newborn children: results from a 13-year incidence study in Arhus, Denmark. Hum Genet 1991;87(1):81–3.
4. Eiben B, Bartels I, Bahr-Porsch S, et al. Cytogenetic analysis of 750 spontaneous abortions with the direct-preparation method of chorionic villi and its implications for studying genetic causes of pregnancy wastage. Am J Hum Genet 1990;47(4): 656–63.
5. Wisniewski A, Milde K, Stupnicki R, et al. Weight deficit at birth and Turner's syndrome. J Pediatr Endocrinol Metab 2007;20(5):607–13.
6. Gil MM, Accurti V, Santacruz B, et al. Analysis of cell-free DNA in maternal blood in screening for aneuploidies: updated meta-analysis. Ultrasound Obstet Gynecol 2017;50(3):302–14.
7. Wolff DJ, Van Dyke DL, Powell CM, Working Group of the ACMG Laboratory Quality Assurance Committee. Laboratory guideline for Turner syndrome. Genet Med 2010;12(1):52–5.
8. Gravholt CH, Fedder J, Naeraa RW, et al. Occurrence of gonadoblastoma in females with Turner syndrome and Y chromosome material: a population study. J Clin Endocrinol Metab 2000;85(9):3199–202.
9. Mortensen KH, Andersen NH, Gravholt CH. Cardiovascular phenotype in Turner syndrome–integrating cardiology, genetics, and endocrinology. Endocr Rev 2012;33(5):677–714.
10. Stochholm K, Juul S, Juel K, et al. Prevalence, incidence, diagnostic delay, and mortality in Turner syndrome. J Clin Endocrinol Metab 2006;91(10):3897–902.
11. Loscalzo ML, Van PL, Ho VB, et al. Association between fetal lymphedema and congenital cardiovascular defects in Turner syndrome. Pediatrics 2005;115(3): 732–5.
12. Clark EB. Neck web and congenital heart defects: a pathogenic association in 45 X-O Turner syndrome? Teratology 1984;29(3):355–61.
13. Bondy CA, Ceniceros I, Van PL, et al. Prolonged rate-corrected QT interval and other electrocardiogram abnormalities in girls with Turner syndrome. Pediatrics 2006;118(4):e1220–1225.
14. Nielsen DG, Nielsen JC, Trolle C, et al. Prolonged QT interval and cardiac arrest after a single dose of amiodarone in a woman with Turner's syndrome. Clin Case Rep 2017;5(2):154–8.
15. Trzcinska D, Olszewska E, Wisniewski A, et al. The knee alignment and the foot arch in patients with Turner syndrome. Pediatr Endocrinol Diabetes Metab 2011;17(3):138–44.
16. Kim JY, Rosenfeld SR, Keyak JH. Increased prevalence of scoliosis in Turner syndrome. J Pediatr Orthop 2001;21(6):765–6.
17. Rappold G, Blum WF, Shavrikova EP, et al. Genotypes and phenotypes in children with short stature: clinical indicators of SHOX haploinsufficiency. J Med Genet 2007;44(5):306–13.

18. Dhooge IJ, De Vel E, Verhoye C, et al. Otologic disease in turner syndrome. Otol Neurotol 2005;26(2):145–50.
19. Trolle C, Hjerrild B, Cleemann L, et al. Sex hormone replacement in Turner syndrome. Endocrine 2012;41(2):200–19.
20. Chellakooty M, Schmidt IM, Haavisto AM, et al. Inhibin A, inhibin B, follicle-stimulating hormone, luteinizing hormone, estradiol, and sex hormone-binding globulin levels in 473 healthy infant girls. J Clin Endocrinol Metab 2003;88(8): 3515–20.
21. Hagen CP, Aksglaede L, Sorensen K, et al. Serum levels of anti-Mullerian hormone as a marker of ovarian function in 926 healthy females from birth to adulthood and in 172 Turner syndrome patients. J Clin Endocrinol Metab 2010;95(11): 5003–10.
22. Sutton EJ, Young J, McInerney-Leo A, et al. Truth-telling and Turner Syndrome: the importance of diagnostic disclosure. J Pediatr 2006;148(1):102–7.
23. Savendahl L, Davenport ML. Delayed diagnoses of Turner's syndrome: proposed guidelines for change. J Pediatr 2000;137(4):455–9.

Mineral Homeostasis and Effects on Bone Mineralization in the Preterm Neonate

Heidi E. Karpen, MD

KEYWORDS

- Calcium • Phosphorus • Parathyroid hormone • Bone mineralization • Bone density
- Rickets of prematurity • Nutrition

KEY POINTS

- Accretion of adequate mineral content in utero is essential for normal bone mineralization.
- Placental mineral transport is accomplished via active transport and does not require fetal hormone input.
- Most mineral accretion occurs during the last trimester of gestation, placing the preterm infant at particular risk for metabolic bone disease.
- Postnatal mineral homeostasis requires a carefully orchestrated balance of actions of parathyroid hormone, calcitonin, and vitamin D on target organs.
- Preterm birth, asphyxia, acidosis, and prolonged parenteral nutrition increase the risk of mineral imbalance and metabolic bone disease.

MINERAL HOMEOSTASIS IN THE FETUS

Mineral accretion by the skeleton before birth depends directly on the adequacy of mineral supply in utero. This mineral supply also regulates the functional activity of the osteoblasts and osteoclasts. Although the bone (through mineral turnover), the intestines, and kidneys are the major source of mineral supply for the adult, the placenta actively transports calcium, phosphorus, and magnesium from the maternal circulation to meet the needs of the growing fetus.

Calcium

The full-term fetus typically accrues approximately 30 g of calcium ($\sim$120–150 mg/kg/d during the third trimester) and up to 300 mg/d during the last month of gestation. Similarly, phosphorus is accrued at rates of approximately 70 mg/kg/d.[1,2]

Because such high levels of mineral concentrations are necessary for normal fetal skeletal development, the placenta is capable of operating against a steep

Pediatrics, Emory University School of Medicine, 2015 Uppergate Drive Northeast, ECC Room 324, Atlanta, GA 30345, USA
E-mail address: heidi.karpen@emory.edu

Clin Perinatol 45 (2018) 129–141
https://doi.org/10.1016/j.clp.2017.11.005
0095-5108/18/© 2017 Elsevier Inc. All rights reserved.

concentration gradient importing calcium via a transcellular, active transport process.[2] This influx of calcium to the fetus is preserved even in circumstances of low mineral concentrations in the maternal circulation caused by severe dietary restriction, vitamin D deficiency, or in more serious conditions, such as combined thyroid/parathyroidectomy or loss of the vitamin D receptor.[3] Animal studies have shown that these high calcium levels are not necessary for survival of the fetus to term but that bones will be undermineralized at birth.[1]

Most (>99%) of the total body calcium stores are associated with hydroxyapatite or other components of collagen and bone matrix or in a noncrystalline calcium phosphate form, whereas less than 1% of the stores are contained in the extracellular fluid (ECF) and soft tissues. Calcium that exists at the edge of the bone mineral crystals is available for exchange with this ECF pool, serving as a ready reservoir for available free calcium.[4] Plasma calcium exists in 3 major forms:

- Free calcium ion (Ca^{2+}) accounts for approximately 50% of the serum calcium pool.
- Calcium is bound to plasma proteins, most of which is albumin, and totals approximately 40% of this pool.
- Diffusible complexes, such as bicarbonate, phosphate, or citrate, account for only approximately 10%.

As the only physiologically active form of calcium in the blood, ionized calcium is integral for many critical cellular functions and is, thus, under tight hormonal regulation, particularly by parathyroid hormone (PTH). It is also subject to acute changes due to blood pH, which decreases protein binding, and the serum albumin concentration, which can affect both the total and ionized calcium levels. Although there is a general correlation between total and ionized calcium levels, this correlation is often poor in neonates. Ca^{2+} balance is maintained via uptake from the intestinal tract, excretion and reabsorption at the kidney, and flux into and out of the bones.

At the time of birth, there is an acute disruption of the maternal-fetal calcium supply. In the absence of an exogenous source of calcium, the infant must increase the flux from bone to the ECF space in order maintain calcium homeostasis and normal serum calcium levels. Calcium levels begin to fall at 2 hours of life and nadir at 24 to 36 hours of age, with more significant declines seen in very-low-birth-weight (VLBW) preterm infants (**Fig. 1**).

The relatively high serum calcium levels in the fetus may also provide protection against neonatal tetany, arrhythmias, and seizures, as these calcium levels decline in the first 48 hours after birth. The deeper nadir seen in preterm infants may be due to gestational unresponsiveness of the parathyroid gland or to uncorrected hypomagnesemia, although hypomagnesemia is not usually associated with tetany or cardiovascular compromise. Interestingly, although serum calcium concentrations at birth are unaffected by sex, race, or weight for gestational age,[5] serum calcium does seem to be affected by mode of delivery (lower for elective caesarean delivery without labor than with labor or for vaginal delivery) and season of birth (lower in summer births than winter births).[6]

Phosphorus

The total body phosphorus in term newborns is approximately 16 g, distributed in a wide array of tissues. In addition to being a primary component of bone, phosphorus plays a major role in almost all metabolic processes through its association with nucleotides in DNA, energy-containing units, such as adenosine-triphosphate, lipid

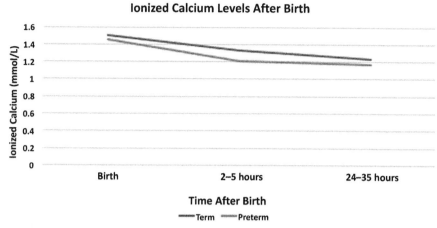

Fig. 1. Serum ionized calcium levels in term and preterm infants after birth. (*Adapted from* Loughead JL, Mimouni F, Tsang RC. Serum ionized calcium concentrations in normal neonates. Am J Dis Child 1988;142(5):516–8; and Wandrup J, Kroner J, Pryds O, et al. Age-related reference values for ionized calcium in the first week of life in premature and full-term neonates. Scand J Clin Lab Invest 1988;48(3):255–60.)

bilayers, and phosphorylation of proteins, controlling their expression and activity. Similar to calcium, most phosphorus (>80%) is accrued during the last trimester of pregnancy at a rate of approximately 75 mg/kg/d and is closely tied to calcium accretion, with a calcium/phosphorus ratio of 1.7:1.0. Similar to calcium, 85% of phosphorus is associated with bone as hydroxyapatite; but the remainder is present in the ECF as inorganic phosphate ions (P_i) and in the intracellular compartment as phosphate esters and intermediates of phosphorylation.

Similar to calcium, serum phosphorus exists as 3 fractions:

- Ionized P_i: approximately 55%
- Protein-bound P_i: a much smaller fraction than calcium, at 11%
- P_i complexed to sodium, calcium, and magnesium: approximately 34%

Phosphorus levels are low immediately after birth, typically about 2.6 mmol/L (range 1.5–3.4 mmol/L), and increase in the first week of life to approximately 3.4 mmol/L. Although not well defined, this phosphorus increase is thought to be due in part to diminished excretion from decreased glomerular filtration rate and to endogenous phosphorus release. In contrast to calcium, serum phosphorus levels at birth do not display differences by sex, race, season of birth, weight for gestational age, or mode of delivery.[6] Serum phosphorus levels are not as tightly regulated as calcium and can vary widely postnatally by diet, age, blood pH, sex, and hormonal influences.

Magnesium

Although magnesium is the second most prevalent divalent cation in the body, it is present in much smaller amounts than both calcium and phosphorus, with a term newborn having a total body magnesium content of approximately 0.8 g. Akin to calcium and phosphorus, magnesium is accrued rapidly during the last trimester of pregnancy at a rate of 3 mg/kg/d.

Most of the magnesium is distributed within tissues, 65% of which is associated with the crystalline component of bone and 34% of which is found in the intracellular space. Only a small fraction of the total magnesium pool is found in the ECF. Magnesium in bone is not a major component of the hydroxyapatite structure but is generally found at the crystal surface. Unlike calcium, only a minor fraction of this is freely exchangeable with extracellular magnesium. Because most of the magnesium is located in tissues, the plasma concentration does not give an accurate measure of total body magnesium content. Stable isotope techniques currently provide the best assessment of the total magnesium pool size.[7]

The plasma fraction of magnesium is present in 3 forms:

- As the free magnesium ion (Mg^+), 55%
- Bound to plasma proteins, such as albumin, 30%
- Complexed to anions, such as phosphate and oxalate, 15%

A significant proportion of the Mg^+ ion is contained in the intracellular cytosolic space and plays a key role in neuromuscular excitability and as a cofactor for many enzymatic reactions. Because of the critical physiologic roles, serum levels of magnesium are tightly regulated and extremely stable, with normal levels of 0.62 to 1.16 mmol/L (1.5–2.8 mg/dL).[8] Large-for-gestational-age infants, infants of diabetic mothers, and preterm infants can show higher serum magnesium levels, that vary inversely with blood pH, similar to calcium.[9]

Ionized magnesium levels can vary significantly in several neonatal conditions, such as respiratory distress syndrome, severe hyperbilirubinemia, and acidosis.[10,11] Although most of the magnesium is as an intracellular cation, serum concentrations may increase because of the extracellular shifts and uncoupling from serum proteins in response to tissue injury, acidosis, and hypoxemia. Magnesium levels are also found to be higher in intrauterine growth restriction preterm infants, although the mechanism of this is not well understood.[12] In contrast, plasma magnesium levels are found to be decreased in asphyxia[13] and during postnatal whole-body cooling, despite repletion and parenteral nutrition (PN).[14] Given the protective effects of magnesium against cellular damage, particularly in the central nervous system, prompt correction is key in these populations in particular.

REGULATION OF CALCIUM AND PHOSPHORUS

The exquisite regulation of serum calcium levels and homeostasis is accomplished primarily through the coordinated interaction of 3 hormones (PTH, calcitonin, and vitamin D) with 3 main target organs: the intestines, kidneys, and bones.

Parathyroid Hormone

PTH is a peptide hormone produced by the parathyroid glands, which are physically adjacent to the thyroid gland. The fetal parathyroid, and to a small degree the fetal thyroid gland, produce PTH; but circulating levels remain low during gestation. Fetal PTH does not seem to play a role in placental transport of calcium. This is illustrated in Hoxa3 −/− mice who do not develop parathyroid glands or secrete PTH but have normal placental calcium transfer with lower-than-normal serum calcium and have bone mineralization defects.[15] Fetal PTH production is likely mediated through the actions of the calcium sensing receptor, which senses high-circulating ionized and total calcium levels provided from the maternal circulation.[1]

Postnatally, a decrease in serum ionized calcium levels triggers production and secretion of PTH into the circulation from the chief cells of the parathyroid gland. PTH then acts through its end organs, the bones, kidneys, and intestines, in a coordinated effort to restore calcium homeostasis (**Fig. 2**). PTH stimulates resorption

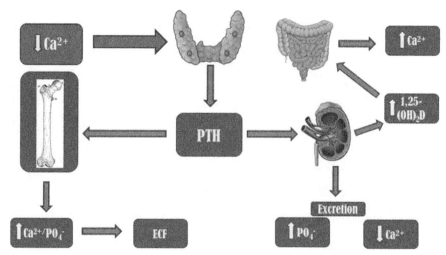

Fig. 2. Response of parathyroid gland to hypocalcemia and the effects on end organs.

of bone by activating osteoclast activity, releasing calcium and phosphorus into the ECF and circulation. PTH concurrently acts on the distal tubule of the kidney to increase urinary excretion of phosphorus and decrease excretion of calcium. PTH also acts to increase production of 1,25 dihydroxyvitamin D (1,25[OH]$_2$D), although this effect requires approximately 24 to 48 hours. Coordination of short and long feedback loops provides the exquisite control of serum calcium levels that are critical for normal homeostasis. Although PTH primarily responds to changes in serum ionized calcium, PTH also has the greatest effect on serum phosphorus concentrations.

Because the fetus experiences a state of relative hypercalcemia via active transport from the placenta, clamping of the umbilical cord at the time of birth causes an acute cessation of this continuous maternal-fetal transport. Serum calcium levels decrease acutely after birth, triggering a 2- to 5-fold increase in PTH levels in the first 48 hours after birth that are sustained for several days. Both term and VLBW preterm infants seem to be able to mount this surge in PTH and respond appropriately, although the nadir in serum calcium for preterm infants may be lower and longer. Serum umbilical PTH levels do not differ by sex, race, weight for age, or season of birth[5,6] but do seem to be higher in elective cesarean delivery without labor (compared with with labor), emergency cesarean delivery, or vaginal delivery.[5] However, the PTH response seems to be blunted in the infant of the diabetic mother and is exacerbated by hypomagnesemia.[16]

Parathyroid Hormone–Related Peptide

PTH-related peptide (PTHrP) is a prohormone that is processed into several circulating peptides in humans, although the physiologic roles of each of these peptide fragments has yet to be elucidated. The PTHrP gene is expressed in numerous tissues of the fetus and placenta, including but not limited to the fetal skeletal growth plates, cardiac and vascular smooth muscle, trophoblasts, intraplacental yolk sac, amnion, chorion, and umbilical cord.[1] Although it seems that both PTH and PTHrP play a role in the maintenance of the fetal blood calcium level (loss of either results in fetal hypocalcemia), loss of both leads to the most severe hypocalcemia.[17]

Because the half-life of PTHrP is quite short, and accurate measurements depend critically on proper sample processing, PTHrP is generally not assessed in routine clinical practice.

Calcitonin

Calcitonin is a peptide hormone produced by the thyroid gland parafollicular cells, which are calcium sensing. Calcitonin increases and decreases in concert with serum calcium levels. Although PTH and calcitonin exert their actions in target organs through distinct molecular pathways, the two hormones work in concert to balance osteoclast-mediated bone resorption and renal calcium and phosphorus excretion. Calcitonin is also secreted in response to elevated serum levels of magnesium and in response to feeding. This response may prevent hypercalcemia after ingestion of calcium-rich foods.[18] Calcitonin is rapidly cleared from the circulation, with a half-life of only 2 to 15 minutes.

Calcitonin is synthesized in both the fetal thyroid and placenta, and the fetal circulating concentration is about twice the maternal level. Umbilical cord levels do not vary by sex, race, or season of birth[6] but decrease with increasing gestation. Calcitonin levels in preterm infants are nearly 3 times those of term infants. Levels of calcitonin increase over the first 2 days of life, declining to childhood levels by the end of the first month of life. This postnatal surge may serve to modulate the calcium resorption induced by increasing levels of PTH after birth.[19]

Vitamin D

Vitamin D enters the body either via absorption from the gastrointestinal tract or via production in the skin in response to ultraviolet light. In order to be used, dietary vitamin D must undergo 2 hydroxylation steps to achieve its active state. The first step, 25-hydroxylation, occurs in the liver and circulating concentrations of 25-hydroxyvitamin D (25-(OH)D) generally reflect the body's vitamin D status from a combination of ingestion and sunlight exposure. In contrast, the second hydroxylation step occurs in the proximal renal tubule, producing the active molecule, calcitriol or 1,25-dihydroxyvitamin D (1,25[OH]$_2$D), a process that is tightly regulated by PTH and by decreased circulating levels of calcium and phosphorus. The activity of 1,25(OH)$_2$D is most akin to a hormone, with 1,25(OH)$_2$D traveling through the circulation to act on target organs in order to achieve its effect of increasing serum calcium levels. The 1,25(OH)$_2$D stimulates absorption of calcium and phosphorus in the small intestine, decreases renal excretion of calcium and phosphorus, decreases bone resorption by osteoclasts, and increases bone maturation and mineralization by osteoblasts and osteocytes (**Fig. 3**).

Circulating fetal calcitriol levels are low, typically 50% of the maternal levels, and are produced by the fetal kidney. Umbilical cord concentrations of 1,25(OH)$_2$D range from 31 to 15 pmol/L and vary by season of birth (being higher in summer-born infants) and by in utero growth restriction but not by sex or race.[6] Levels of 1,25(OH)$_2$D are low at birth but rapidly increase to normal adult levels by 24 hours of life. In contrast, preterm infants have serum 1,25(OH)$_2$D levels that are more comparable with adult levels and continue to increase over the first few months of life, often to levels 4 to 6 times that seen in term neonates.[1] These low concentrations in utero are likely due to suppression of calcitriol synthesis by a combination of high serum calcium and phosphorus levels and low PTH levels, coupled with increased activity of the catabolic enzyme 24-hydroxylase.

As opposed to 1,25(OH)$_2$D, umbilical cord concentrations of 25-(OH)D are influenced by season of birth, being nearly 50% lower in winter (parallels sunshine

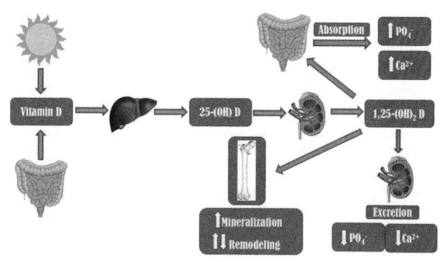

Fig. 3. Processing and activity of vitamin D.

exposure), and are a better reflection of maternal vitamin D status as 25-(OH)D readily crosses the placenta. Prenatal vitamins blunt the effect of season and sunshine exposure on the 25-(OH)D concentrations at birth, which positively affects bone mineralization in the fetus. Interestingly, although the loss of either PTH or PTHrP causes fetal hypocalcemia and hyperphosphatemia, the loss of calcitonin or 25-(OH)D or 1,25(OH)$_2$D or the vitamin D receptor causes no change in fetal serum mineral concentration.[1]

BONE MINERALIZATION DISORDERS
Rickets

The term *rickets* denotes an undermineralized skeleton usually associated with deficiency of calcium or phosphorus accretion in the bone. A key element to the differential diagnosis is timing of this undermineralization. A rachitic-appearing fetal skeleton suggests congenital rickets that is most often due to skeletal dysplasias, osteogenesis imperfecta, metaphyseal chondrodysplasias, fetal hypoparathyroidism, or hypophosphatasia syndromes, which are beyond the scope of this article.

Neither maternal nutritional deficiencies nor vitamin D deficiency alone are sufficient to cause undermineralization of the fetal skeleton, except in cases of severe malnutrition, untreated pancreatic insufficiency, combined vitamin D/calcium/phosphorus depletion, or use of medications that interfere with vitamin D metabolism.[1] Exposure of the fetus prenatally to magnesium (as prevention for preterm birth and as neuroprotection) has been associated with particularly poor bone mineralization and congenital rickets,[20] especially in the setting of multiple gestations.

Rickets of Prematurity

Normal skeletal formation and bone mineralization in the fetus is a process that depends on the actions of PTH and PTHrP and on provision of adequate mineral content from the maternal circulation. In contrast to their effects on calcium and phosphorus homeostasis, calcitonin, calcitriol, and sex steroids are not essential to this process.[1]

Given sufficient accretion of mineral content, and absence of any genetic bone mineralization disorders, the fetal skeleton will attain its full bone mass potential. However, most of the mineral accretion occurs, in the last trimester of pregnancy, leaving preterm infants in the precarious position of missing most of this critical accumulation.

The inability of most VLBW infants to tolerate significant enteral feedings, the low mineral content of human milk (HM), and inadequate provision of minerals in most PN preparations predispose preterm infants for metabolic bone disease (MBD). MBD of prematurity is associated with decreased organic protein bone matrix (osteopenia) and/or decreased mineral deposition (osteomalacia). Osteopenia and osteomalacia can exist in isolation or in combination and may be associated with rachitic changes.

Chronic diseases, such as bronchopulmonary dysplasia, necrotizing enterocolitis, and patent ductus arteriosus, lead to decreased mineral intake through prolonged PN intake and slow advancement of fully fortified enteral feedings and fluid restriction coupled with diuretic and steroid use (further limiting and wasting mineral content). This chronic deficiency of calcium and phosphorus at a time of rapid neonatal growth leads to physical and radiologic signs of rickets of prematurity, beginning with osteopenia, metaphyseal flaring, and widening of the epiphyses of long bones and eventually progressing to rachitic rosary and pathologic fractures particularly in the rib, femur, and humerus. Improvements in neonatal care and nutrition since the 1980s have led to a marked decrease in the overall incidence of MBD of prematurity, but survival of smaller infants born at earlier gestational ages continues to provide challenges for bone health.

A recent retrospective cohort study of extremely low-birth-weight infants showed a 30% incidence of MBD of prematurity, with nearly 34% of infants with MBD developing spontaneous fractures. These infants were more likely to be of lower birth weight, more premature, and with higher severity of illness. Concomitant with these characteristics, these infants were more likely to have longer courses of mechanical ventilation and a higher incidence of chronic lung disease and had higher exposure to diuretics, postnatal steroids, and antibiotics.[21] A retrospective review of VLBW infants pointed to longer courses of PN and higher direct bilirubin levels in infants who developed MBD.[22] PN is often not formulated to deliver the recommended 150 mg/kg/d calcium and 75 mg/kg/d phosphorus that a growing preterm infant requires because of the fluid volume constraints and inadequate provision of protein. Aluminum contamination of PN has also been cited as a factor contributing to MBD and is a persistent issue in common PN preparations.[23,24]

Elevated alkaline phosphatase (ALP) levels have been associated with MBD of prematurity, often predicting poor linear growth in childhood.[25] The suggested cutoff values for serum ALP range from 500 IU/L to as high as 1200 IU/L in older studies.[26–29] The use of serum phosphorus levels (in addition to serum ALP) increases sensitivity and specificity for the detection of MBD of prematurity.[30] It is clear from the myriad of studies on this topic that no single value of ALP reliably predicts radiological findings of rickets.[31] Hence, a practice of routine ALP screening coupled with serum phosphorus levels is key for early recognition and treatment of MBD of prematurity. Skeletal films, speed of sound ultrasound, and dual-energy x-ray absorptiometry may also be used as adjuvants to diagnose osteopenia, clinical rickets, and fractures.[32,33]

NUTRITIONAL SUPPORT

As outlined earlier, these fragile preterm infants are born significantly disadvantaged from a mineral accretion standpoint. Fortunately, the neonatal intestine has a nearly insaturable capacity for mineral absorption. Several studies have shown that calcium absorption in neonates is proportional to intake and does not depend on vitamin D intake, as opposed to calcium absorption in older infants and children. This passive absorption of calcium allows preterm infants (who are able to tolerate enteral feeds) to absorb all of the calcium and phosphorus offered to them.[34] It is important to emphasize that sufficient serum phosphorus concentrations, in addition to calcium, are key for normal bone mineralization. Vitamin D may not play a key role in mineral absorption early on in preterm infants, but it is not clear when in infancy this begins to play a more substantial role. In the absence of severe renal disease or vitamin D–resistant rickets, vitamin D status should be monitored using 25-(OH)D, as this is the best assessment of nutritional vitamin D sufficiency.[35]

Essential to the prevention of MBD, and nitrogen deficit often seen in the VLBW preterm infant, is the provision of early aggressive PN with adequate protein and mineral content.[36] Newer crystalloid amino acid mixtures avoid issues of hyperammonemia, acidosis, and uremia that plagued early attempts at neonatal PN.[37] Protein and minerals (particularly calcium and phosphorus) are coupled in PN, as both are needed to modulate the pH and solubility of the PN solution.[24] Without adequate protein, approximately 3.5 to 4.0 g/kg/d, it is impossible to meet the minimum goal of 150 mg/kg/d of calcium and 75 mg/kg/d of phosphorus (mimicking in utero protein and mineral accretion rates for the last trimester of gestation).[38] Prompt provision of optimal PN halts the nitrogen deficit and bone resorption that occur in early postnatal days and allows for accretion and growth to continue.[39]

Initiation of enteral feedings is typically begun with HM, ideally mother's own milk (MOM)[40] or pasteurized donor HM when MOM supply is insufficient.[41] Although HM is the ideal source of nutrition for all neonates and infants, some nurseries do not have access or cannot afford donor breast milk and must resort to formula use. HM alone is insufficient to provide adequate protein and mineral content and is associated with lower bone mineralization in preterm infants.[38] The American Academy of Pediatrics Committee on Nutrition recommends 150 to 220 mg/kg/d of calcium, 75 to 140 mg/kg/d of phosphorus, and 200 to 400 IU/d of vitamin D for enterally fed VLBW infants.[35] Fully fortified HM and specialized preterm formulas are designed to provide adequate protein, calcium, phosphorus, and vitamin D content to meet the needs of the growing preterm infant for growth and mineral accretion during this period of rapid growth (**Table 1**).

The use of fortified HM or preterm formula is recommended for infants less than 1800 g to 2000 g, without specific gestational age correlates, because small-for-gestational-age infants have a greater risk of MBD and nutritional deficiencies than age-matched appropriate-for-gestational age infants.[42] The use of these highly fortified products is recommended at least until the infant reaches the equivalent of 36 weeks' gestational age and/or 2000 g before beginning the change to unfortified HM, preferably breastfeeding, or term formula (see **Table 1**). Transitional formulas contain an intermediate amount of protein and mineral content (between that provided in preterm formula or fortified HM and term formula or unfortified HM) and may be indicated in some high-risk infants, although recent Cochrane reviews suggest that the effects on growth and neurodevelopmental outcomes are minimal.[43,44] Infants who have had prolonged courses of PN, are fluid restricted, or who have elevated ALP may benefit from continuing on fully fortified HM or preterm formula until closer to hospital discharge. Fully fortified products typically contain sufficient vitamin D to meet the needs of a growing preterm infant, but the addition of vitamin D is recommended (200 IU/d in formula-fed infants and 400 IU/d in HM-fed infants) when they reach 2000 g or are approaching discharge. Continued surveillance of growth, and in some cases metabolic parameters, is key to the long-term outcomes of VLBW infants after they transition to home.

Table 1
Composition of mature human milk, bovine and human milk–based fortified human milk, preterm and transitional formulas (per 100 calories)

	Mature HM	Fortified HM (Bovine Fortifier)[a]	Fortified HM (Donor Milk Fortifier +4)[b]	Preterm Formula[a,c]	Transitional Formula[a,c]	Term Formula[a,c]
Energy (kcal)	65–70	100	100	100	~74	~68
Protein (g)	1.03	4.0	2.8	3.0–3.6	2.1	1.4–1.5
Carbohydrate (g)	6.7–7.0	8.1	8.7	~10.5	7.5–7.9	~7.5
Fat (g)	3.5	6.0	5.98	5.0–5.4	3.9–4.1	3.4–3.8
Calcium (mg)	20–25	145	150	165–180	78–89	45–53
Phosphorus	12–14	80	78	90–100	46–49	25–29
Sodium (mg)	12–25	57	70	43–70	~25	16–18
Iron (mg)	0.3–0.9	1.91	0.24	1.8	~1.3	1.0–1.2

[a] Mead Johnson Nutritionals: http://www.meadjohnson.com.
[b] Prolacta Bioscience: http://www/.prolacta.com/human-milk-fortifier-1.
[c] Abbott Nutrition, Abbott Laboratories: http://abbottnutrition.com.

SUMMARY

Active placental transport provides the fetus with adequate mineral accretion, except in cases of extreme nutritional deprivation of the mother, and does not require fetal hormonal input. Most of this accretion occurs during the third trimester of gestation, placing the smallest preterm infants at greatest risk for MBD. Neonatal conditions, such as chronic lung disease, acidosis, and cholestasis, and exposure to medications, such as steroids and diuretics, alter mineral deposition and increase excretion. The provision of adequate protein, calories, and mineral content through early aggressive PN and fortified enteral products is key to the prevention and treatment of MBD in the preterm infant.

Best Practices

What is the current practice?

Metabolic bone disease of the preterm infant

Nutritional practices vary widely by institution across the country and world. Many clinicians are wary about early provision of adequate protein because of fears of hyperammonemia, acidosis, and uremia and, thus, limit mineral content in parenteral nutrition. Concerns for potential NEC often delays fortification of HM or moving to full-strength preterm formula.

What changes in current practice are likely to improve outcomes?

Major recommendations

Provision of early aggressive PN in the first days after birth
- At least 3.5 to 4.0 g/kg/d protein, 150 to 200 mg/kg/d calcium, 75 to 90 mg/kg/d phosphorus
- Move to fully fortified HM or full-strength preterm formula as soon as feasible
- Screening calcium, phosphorus, and ALP every 1 to 2 weeks
- Consider long bone and chest films to screen for fractures if ALP greater than 500 to 700 IU/L
- Continue fortified HM or preterm formula until infant is 1800 g to 2000 g

Rating for the strength of the evidence: strong

Bibliographic sources: see reference section

Summary statement

Most mineral accretion occurs in the last trimester of gestation, placing preterm infants at particular risk for MBD. Early, aggressive nutrition is key to the prevention and treatment of MBD.

REFERENCES

1. Kovacs CS. Bone development and mineral homeostasis in the fetus and neonate: roles of the calciotropic and phosphotropic hormones. Physiol Rev 2014;94(4):1143–218.
2. Mitchell DM, Jüppner H. Regulation of calcium homeostasis and bone metabolism in the fetus and neonate. Curr Opin Endocrinol Diabetes Obes 2010; 17(1):25–30.
3. Kovacs CS. Calcium, phosphorus, and bone metabolism in the fetus and newborn. Early Hum Dev 2015;91(11):623–8.
4. Abrams SA, Esteban NV, Vieira NE, et al. Developmental changes in calcium kinetics in children assessed using stable isotopes. J Bone Miner Res 1992;7(3): 287–93.
5. Bagnoli F, Bruchi S, Garosi G, et al. Relationship between mode of delivery and neonatal calcium homeostasis. Eur J Pediatr 1990;149(11):800–3.
6. Namgung R, Tsang RC, Specker BL, et al. Low bone mineral content and high serum osteocalcin and 1,25-dihydroxyvitamin D in summer- versus winter-born newborn infants: an early fetal effect? J Pediatr Gastroenterol Nutr 1994;19(2): 220–7.
7. Coudray C, Feillet-Coudray C, Rambeau M, et al. Stable isotopes in studies of intestinal absorption, exchangeable pools and mineral status: the example of magnesium. J Trace Elem Med Biol 2005;19(1):97–103.
8. Handwerker SM, Altura BT, Royo B, et al. Ionized serum magnesium levels in umbilical cord blood of normal pregnant women at delivery: relationship to calcium, demographics, and birthweight. Am J Perinatol 1993;10(5):392–7.
9. Mehta R, Petrova A. Ionized magnesium and gestational age. Indian J Pediatr 2007;74(11):1025–8.
10. Olofsson K, Matthiesen G, Rudnicki M. Whole blood ionized magnesium in neonatal acidosis and preterm infants: a prospective consecutive study. Acta Paediatr 2001;90(12):1398–401.
11. Sarici SU, Serdar MA, Erdem G, et al. Evaluation of plasma ionized magnesium levels in neonatal hyperbilirubinemia. Pediatr Res 2004;55(2):243–7.
12. Barbosa NOE, Okay TS, Leone CR. Magnesium and intrauterine growth restriction. J Am Coll Nutr 2005;24(1):10–5.
13. Khalessi N, Mazouri A, Bassirnia M, et al. Comparison between serum magnesium levels of asphyxiated neonates and normal cases. Med J Islam Repub Iran 2017;31(1):19–112.
14. Tocco NM, Hodge AE, Jones AA, et al. Neonatal therapeutic hypothermia-associated hypomagnesemia during parenteral nutrition therapy. Nutr Clin Pract 2014;29(2):246–8.
15. Miao D, He B, Karaplis AC, et al. Parathyroid hormone is essential for normal fetal bone formation. J Clin Invest 2002;109(9):1173–82.
16. Mimouni F, Loughead JL, Tsang RC, et al. Postnatal surge in serum calcitonin concentrations: no contribution to neonatal hypocalcemia in infants of diabetic mothers. Pediatr Res 1990;28(5):493–5.
17. Ohata Y, Ozono K, Michigami T. Current concepts in perinatal mineral metabolism. Clin Pediatr Endocrinol 2016;25(1):9–17.
18. Pedrazzoni M, Ciotti G, Davoli L, et al. Meal-stimulated gastrin release and calcitonin secretion. J Endocrinol Invest 1989;12(6):409–12.

19. Venkataraman PS, Tsang RC, Chen IW, et al. Pathogenesis of early neonatal hypocalcemia: studies of serum calcitonin, gastrin, and plasma glucagon. J Pediatr 1987;110(4):599–603.

20. Lamm CI, Norton KI, Murphy RJ, et al. Congenital rickets associated with magnesium sulfate infusion for tocolysis. J Pediatr 1988;113(6):1078–82.

21. Viswanathan S, Khasawneh W, McNelis K, et al. Metabolic bone disease: a continued challenge in extremely low birth weight infants. JPEN J Parenter Enteral Nutr 2014;38(8):982–90.

22. Ukarapong S, Venkatarayappa SKB, Navarrete C, et al. Risk factors of metabolic bone disease of prematurity. Early Hum Dev 2017;112:29–34.

23. Fanni D, Ambu R, Gerosa C, et al. Aluminum exposure and toxicity in neonates: a practical guide to halt aluminum overload in the prenatal and perinatal periods. World J Pediatr 2014;10(2):101–7.

24. Boullata JI, Gilbert K, Sacks G, et al. A.S.P.E.N. clinical guidelines: parenteral nutrition ordering, order review, compounding, labeling, and dispensing. JPEN J Parenter Enteral Nutr 2014;38(3):334–77.

25. Rover MMS, Viera CS, Silveira RC, et al. Risk factors associated with growth failure in the follow-up of very low birth weight newborns. J Pediatr (Rio J) 2016; 92(3):307–13.

26. Lucas A, Brooke OG, Baker BA, et al. High alkaline phosphatase activity and growth in preterm neonates. Arch Dis Child 1989;64(7 Spec No):902–9.

27. Mitchell SM, Rogers SP, Hicks PD, et al. High frequencies of elevated alkaline phosphatase activity and rickets exist in extremely low birth weight infants despite current nutritional support. BMC Pediatr 2009;9(1):47.

28. Abdallah EAA, Said RN, Mosallam DS, et al. Serial serum alkaline phosphatase as an early biomarker for osteopenia of prematurity. Medicine (Baltimore) 2016; 95(37):e4837.

29. Figueras-Aloy J, Álvarez-Domínguez E, Pérez-Fernández JM, et al. Metabolic bone disease and bone mineral density in very preterm infants. J Pediatr 2014; 164(3):499–504.

30. Backström MC, Kouri T, Kuusela AL, et al. Bone isoenzyme of serum alkaline phosphatase and serum inorganic phosphate in metabolic bone disease of prematurity. Acta Paediatr 2000;89(7):867–73.

31. Faerk J, Peitersen B, Petersen S, et al. Bone mineralisation in premature infants cannot be predicted from serum alkaline phosphatase or serum phosphate. Arch Dis Child Fetal Neonatal Ed 2002;87(2):F133–6.

32. Longhi S, Mercolini F, Carloni L, et al. Prematurity and low birth weight lead to altered bone geometry, strength, and quality in children. J Endocrinol Invest 2015;38(5):563–8.

33. Mercy J, Dillon B, Morris J, et al. Relationship of tibial speed of sound and lower limb length to nutrient intake in preterm infants. Arch Dis Child Fetal Neonatal Ed 2007;92(5):F381–5.

34. Kovacs CS. Bone metabolism in the fetus and neonate. Pediatr Nephrol 2014; 29(5):793–803.

35. Abrams SA, Committee on Nutrition. Calcium and vitamin d requirements of enterally fed preterm infants. Pediatrics 2013;131(5):e1676–83.

36. Denne SC, Poindexter BB. Evidence supporting early nutritional support with parenteral amino acid infusion. Semin Perinatol 2007;31(2):56–60.

37. ElHassan NO, Kaiser JR. Parenteral nutrition in the neonatal intensive care unit. Neoreviews 2011;12(3):e130–40.

38. Nehra D, Carlson SJ, Fallon EM, et al. A.S.P.E.N. clinical guidelines: nutrition support of neonatal patients at risk for metabolic bone disease. JPEN J Parenter Enteral Nutr 2013;37(5):570–98.
39. Pereira-da-Silva L, Costa AB, Pereira L, et al. Early high calcium and phosphorus intake by parenteral nutrition prevents short-term bone strength decline in preterm infants. J Pediatr Gastroenterol Nutr 2011;52(2):203–9.
40. Section on Breastfeeding. Breastfeeding and the use of human milk. Pediatrics 2012;129(3):e827–41.
41. Committee on Nutrition, Section on Breastfeeding, Committee on Fetus and Newborn. Donor human milk for the high-risk infant: preparation, safety, and usage options in the United States. Pediatrics 2017;139(1):e20163440.
42. Lapillonne A, Braillon P, Claris O, et al. Body composition in appropriate and in small for gestational age infants. Acta Paediatr 1997;86(2):196–200.
43. Young L, Embleton ND, McGuire W. Nutrient-enriched formula versus standard formula for preterm infants following hospital discharge. Cochrane Database Syst Rev 2016;(12):CD004696.
44. Young L, Embleton ND, McCormick FM, et al. Multinutrient fortification of human breast milk for preterm infants following hospital discharge. Cochrane Database Syst Rev 2013;(2):CD004866.

Appendices A to C

APPENDIX A. NEONATAL ADRENAL INSUFFICIENCY—RECENT PUBLICATIONS
Outline by Susan R. Rose, MD

Guran T, Buonocore F, Saka N, et al. Rare causes of primary adrenal insufficiency: genetic and clinical characterization of a large nationwide cohort. J Clin Endocrinol Metab 2016;101:284–92.

Primary adrenal insufficiency (PAI) is a life-threatening condition often due to monogenic causes in children.

Objective: Clinical characteristics and molecular genetics of children with PAI were investigated.

Structured questionnaire at 19 tertiary pediatric endocrinology clinics, followed by genetic analysis, was performed using HaloPlex capture and next-generation sequencing in 95 children (48 girls, aged 0–18 years, 8 familial). Children with congenital adrenal hyperplasia (CAH) were excluded.

Results: Genetic diagnosis in 77 patients (81%) included MC2R (n = 25), NR0B1 (n = 12), STAR (n = 11), CYP11A1 (n = 9), MRAP (n = 9), NNT (n = 7), ABCD1 (n = 2), NR5A1 (n = 1), and AAAS (n = 1).

Mutations occurred in several genes, such as c.560delT in MC2R, p.R451W in CYP11A1, and c.IVS3ds+1delG in MRAP.

Conclusion: Achieving a molecular diagnosis in more than 80% of children has important impact for counseling families, presymptomatic diagnosis, personalized treatment (eg, mineralocorticoid replacement), and predicting comorbidities (eg, neurologic puberty or fertility).

Osuwannaratana P, Nimkarn S, Santiprabhob J, et al. The etiologies of adrenal insufficiency in 73 Thai children: 20 years experience. J Med Assoc Thai 2008;91:1544–50.

Background: Adrenal insufficiency (AI) is the inadequate secretion or action of adrenal hormones (primary or first-degree, secondary or second-degree), resulting in morbidity and mortality when undiagnosed or ineffectively treated.

Retrospective analysis of data of children with AI was conducted between 1982 and 2002 (20 years).

Results: AI was diagnosed in 73 children (42 girls), 62 (84.9%) with first-degree AI and 11 (15.1%) with second-degree AI.

First-degree
- 87.1% had CAH
- 4.8% corticotropin unresponsiveness
- 8.1% had no definite diagnosis
- Common presentation included hyperpigmentation.

Second-degree AI
- 63.6% had panhypopituitarism
- 9.1% isolated corticotropin deficiency
- 27.3% had low birth weight.

Conclusion: CAH was the most common cause of first-degree AI. Panhypopituitarism was the most common cause of second-degree AI, with other causes of AI being rare.

Clin Perinatol 45 (2018) 143–153
https://doi.org/10.1016/j.clp.2017.11.006
0095-5108/18/

Bizzarri C, Olivini N, Pedicelli S, et al. *Congenital primary adrenal insufficiency and selective aldosterone defects presenting as salt-wasting in infancy: a single center 10-year experience. Ital J Pediatr 2016;42:73.*

Salt-wasting represents an emergency in infants, with potential life-threatening complications. Renal function in the neonate is immature with low glomerular filtration rate and reduced ability to concentrate urine.

Retrospective chart review for infants hospitalized with hyponatremia (serum sodium <130 mEq/L) was conducted at a single institution, from 2006 through 2015.

Results: Of 51 infants identified, 19 (37.3%) had CAH, 13 (25.5%) had non-CAH salt-wasting forms of adrenal origin, 10 (19.6%) had central nervous system diseases, and 9 (17.6%) had chronic gastrointestinal or renal salt losses or reduced sodium intake.

CAH type was 21-hydroxylase deficiency in 18, and 3β-hydroxysteroid dehydrogenase (3βHSD) deficiency in 1.

Familial X-linked adrenal hypoplasia congenital (NROB1 gene mutation) were identified in 4.

Aldosterone synthase deficiency (CYP11B2 gene mutation) was identified in 2.

Familial glucocorticoid deficiency (MC2R gene mutations) was identified in 2. Pseudohypoaldosteronism (mutations of the SCNN1G gene encoding for the epithelial sodium channel) was identified in 1.

Two with renal malformations had transient pseudohypoaldosteronism.

An etiologic factor was not identified in 2.

Conclusion: Emergency management of infants with hyponatremia or salt wasting (SW) requires
- Correction of water losses
- Treatment of electrolyte imbalances
- A blood sample for hormonal investigations (should be collected before starting steroid therapy)
- A blood sample to address the analysis of candidate genes.

Flück CE, Pandey AV, Dick B, et al. *Characterization of novel StAR (steroidogenic acute regulatory protein) mutations causing non-classic lipoid adrenal hyperplasia. PLoS One 2011;6:e20178.*

Steroidogenic acute regulatory protein (StAR) is involved in transporting cholesterol to mitochondria for biosynthesis of steroids. Loss of StAR function causes lipoid CAH.

The goal was to provide clinical, biochemical, genetic, protein structure, and functional data on 2 novel StAR mutations.

Two infants with AI in a nonconsanguineous white family
- AI identified in girl at age of 10 months of age and in boy at 14 months
- Normal external genitalia, normal puberty, no signs of hypergonadotropic hypogonadism at age 32 years in girl and at age 29 years in boy.

Results: StAR gene analysis resulted in 2 novel compound heterozygote mutations T44HfsX3 (loss-of-function mutation), and G221S (retains partial activity, ~30%).

Conclusion: StAR mutations in the cholesterol-binding pocket (V187M, R188C, R192C, G221D/S) seem to cause nonclassic lipoid CAH.

Tajima T, Fukushi M. Neonatal mass screening for 21-hydroxylase deficiency. Clin Pediatr Endocrinol 2016;25:1–8.

CAH is due to 21-hydroxylase deficiency:
- Inherited autosomal recessive AI
- Incidence 1 in 10,000 to 20,000 worldwide
- Three forms: SW, simple virilizing, and nonclassic.

SW is the most severe:
- Presents in the first months of life with life-threatening AI
- Potential wrong gender assignment of 46,XX female patients with SW.

Neonatal mass screening of 17-hydroxyprogesterone (17OHP) is performed in several countries, including Japan:
- Positive predictive value (PPV) remains low, especially in preterm (PT) infants.

Second-tier testing with liquid chromatography with tandem mass spectrometry may be useful in reducing false-positive rate and increasing PPV.

Gruñieiro-Papendieck L, Chiesa A, Mendez V, et al. Neonatal screening for congenital adrenal hyperplasia: experience and results in Argentina. J Pediatr Endocrinol Metab 2008;21:73–8.

Results of neonatal screening for CAH were reported in Buenos Aires, Argentina, from 1997 to 2006.

Methods: 17OHP was measured with immunofluorometric assay in filter paper blood samples collected at neonatal maternity discharge:
- Less than 40 nmol/L were normal
- 40 to 90 nmol/L triggered repeat assessment
- Greater than 90 nmol/L confirmed CAH
- Normal was adjusted for gestational age and/or birth weight.

Results were reported from 80,436 screened newborns (46.8% girls), 8848 (11%) were PT:
- 15 term (T) and 3 PT infants were recalled (0.022%)
- 9 were confirmed with CAH (8 T and 1 PT; girl or boy: 0.8; incidence 1:8937)
- Mean ages of screening and treatment were 5.7 and 13 days
- Only 33% were clinically suspected of having CAH before screening
- 4 boys and 2 girls presented salt-wasting forms
- Severe AI crises were prevented as result of screening.

Conclusion: CAH neonatal screening was beneficial, with high incidence of the classic form. Screening allowed detection of unrecognized affected boys and girls, and prevention of salt-wasting crises.

Falhammar H, Wedell A, Nordenström A. Biochemical and genetic diagnosis of 21-hydroxylase deficiency. Endocrine 2015;50:306–14.

Classic CAH due to 21-hydroxylase deficiency
- Caused by mutations in the CYP21A2 gene
- 17OHP level greater than 300 nmol/L
- Often fatal in its classic forms if not treated with glucocorticoids.

Nonclassic CAH (NCCAH)
- Prevalence from 0.1% to 5% in certain ethnicities
- Mild partial cortisol insufficiency
- Survival without treatment.

Most NCCAH patients are never identified but they may have hyperandrogenism, especially female patients:
- 17OHP level 30 to 300 nmol/L in adult men or women (follicular phase or if anovulatory) indicates NCCAH
- Gold standard for diagnosing NCCAH is the corticotropin stimulation test.

The most common CYP21A2 mutations are deletion, large gene conversions, and 9 microconversion-derived mutations. In addition, about 200 rare mutations have been described.

Neonatal screening for CAH
- Main goal of reducing mortality and morbidity due to salt-losing adrenal crises in the newborn period
- Shorten the time to diagnosis in virilized girls
- Misses milder classic CAH and most NCCAH cases.

Conclusion: Diagnosing classic CAH is life-saving but diagnosing NCCAH is also important to prevent unnecessary suffering.

APPENDIX B. NEONATAL MICROBIOME AND ENDOCRINE EFFECTS—RECENT PUBLICATIONS

Yang I, Corwin EJ, Brennan PA, et al. The infant microbiome: implications for infant health and neurocognitive development. Nurs Res 2016;65:76–88.

Beginning at birth, gut microbes participate in digestion and metabolism of food, activation of the immune system, and production of neurotransmitters affecting behavior and cognition.

Factors known to affect the composition of the infant microbiome include
- Mode of delivery (vaginal vs surgical)
- Antibiotic exposure
- Infant-feeding patterns

The gut microbiome influences
- Immunology
- Endocrine system
- Neural pathways

It plays an important role in infant physical and neurocognitive development and lifecourse disease risk.

Keunen K, van Elburg RM, van Bel F, et al. Impact of nutrition on brain development and its neuroprotective implications following preterm birth. Pediatr Res 2015;77:148–55.

Nutrition has important effects on brain development in PT infants.

Early nutrient intake influences brain growth and maturation:
- Effects persist into childhood and adolescence.

Progression of white matter injury caused by inflammation is the most common pattern of brain injury in PT infants.

Nutritional components with immunomodulatory and/or antiinflammatory effects may be neuroprotective. Neuroprotection may result from use of probiotics, prebiotic oligosaccharides, and certain amino acids. The amino acid glutamine may decrease infectious morbidity in PT infants.

Conclusion: Early postnatal nutrition is of major importance for brain growth and maturation. Nutritional components might play a neuroprotective role against white matter injury (through modulation of inflammation and infection) and may influence the microbiome-gut-brain axis.

Cacho N, Neu J. Manipulation of the intestinal microbiome in newborn infants. Adv Nutr 2014;5:114–8.

The gastrointestinal tract harbors a diverse microbial population (the microbiome) affecting
- Nutrition
- Metabolism
- Protection against pathogens
- Development of the immune system.

Development of the intestinal microbiome (at least 1000 different bacterial species)
- Often begins before birth
- Affected by environmental factors, including premature delivery, mode of delivery, antibiotic usage, and diet
- Disturbance in the microbiome during fetal life or the perinatal period may result in adverse consequences.

Cong X, Xu W, Romisher R, et al. Gut microbiome and infant health: brain-gut-microbiota axis and host genetic factors. Yale J Biol Med 2016;89:299–308.

Neonatal gut microbiome is influenced by multiple factors:
- Delivery mode
- Feeding
- Medication use
- Hospital environment
- Early life stress
- Genetics.

Abnormal balance of gut microbiota persists through infancy, especially in high-risk PT infants. Role of the gut microbiome in brain-gut signaling system, and its interaction with host genetics affect short-term and long-term infant health. Further research is needed regarding the brain-gut-microbiota signaling system and the host-microbial interaction in the regulation of health, stress response, and development in human newborns.

Cong X, Henderson WA, Graf J, et al. Early life experience and gut microbiome: the brain-gut-microbiota signaling system. Adv Neonatal Care 2015;15:314–23.

Ongoing advances in neonatal care have led to substantial increases in survival among PT infants. Recent concerns include
- Interplay between stressful early-life experiences and the immature neuroimmune systems
- Brain-gut signaling system.

Microbial species, ligands, and/or products within the developing intestine play a key role:
- Early programming of the central nervous system
- Regulation of intestinal innate immunity.

Understanding of these relationships will potentially lead to changes in practice and targeted interventions.

Gülden E, Wong FS, Wen L. The gut microbiota and type 1 diabetes. Clin Immunol 2015;159:143–53.

Type 1 diabetes mellitus (T1DM)
- Multifactorial
- Immune-mediated disease

- Progressive destruction of autologous insulin-producing beta cells in the pancreas
- Risk affected by genetic, epigenetic, and environmental factors
- Rising incidence cannot be explained by genetic factors alone.

Lifestyle changes (diet, hygiene, and antibiotic usage) may contribute to this rising T1DM incidence.

Gut microbiota are affected by all these factors.

There is a need to design new microbiota-based therapies in the prevention and treatment of T1DM.

Virtanen SM, Takkinen HM, Nwaru BI, et al. Microbial exposure in infancy and subsequent appearance of type 1 diabetes mellitus-associated autoantibodies: a cohort study. JAMA Pediatr 2014;168:755–63.

Role of perinatal microbial exposure in development of T1DM is unclear.

Objective: Investigate whether animal contact and other microbial exposures during infancy alter development of clinical T1DM.

Birth cohort of children with HLA-DQB1-conferred susceptibility to T1DM

- 3143 consecutively born children, 1996 to 2004.

Exposures during year 1 of life were tracked

- Indoor and outdoor dogs, cats, and farm animals
- Farming
- Visit to a stable
- Day care
- Exposure to antibiotics during the first week of life.

Outcomes: Clinical and preclinical T1DM (positivity for islet-cell antibodies plus for other diabetes-associated autoantibodies). Autoantibodies were analyzed at 3-month to 12-month intervals after birth of the child.

Results: Children exposed to an indoor dog had reduced odds of

- Preclinical T1DM (adjusted odds ratio [OR] 0.47, 95% CI 0.28–0.80, $P = .005$)
- Clinical T1DM (adjusted OR 0.40, 95% CI 0.14–1.14, $P = .08$).

The other microbial exposures had no association with preclinical or clinical diabetes.

In conclusion, indoor dog exposure during year 1 of life was inversely associated with preclinical T1DM.

Kimpimäki T, Kupila A, Hämäläinen AM, et al. The first signs of beta-cell autoimmunity appear in infancy in genetically susceptible children from the general population: the Finnish type 1 diabetes prediction and prevention study. J Clin Endocrinol Metab 2001;86:4782–8.

Factors contributing to preclinical T1DM during the first years of life are not yet confirmed. Prospective birth cohort study evaluated

- Appearance of diabetes-associated autoantibodies as a sign of beta-cell autoimmunity
- Development of T1DM.

Of 25,983 newborn infants, 2448 genetically susceptible children were monitored for islet cell antibodies (ICAs) at 3-month to 6-month intervals.

In infants seroconverting to ICA positivity, samples were also analyzed for autoantibodies to

- Insulin (IAA)

- The 65-kDa isoform of glutamic acid decarboxylase
- The protein tyrosine phosphatase-related IA-2 molecule.

Results:

- 15 of those with high-risk genotype (2.7%) and 23 of those with moderate-risk genotype (1.2%, $P = .019$) tested positive for ICA at least once
- 25 of the 38 showed positivity for 2 + antibodies
- IAA appeared first in 22 of the 38 ($P<.019$ or less)
- First autoantibodies appeared in most in the fall and winter (30 of 38 vs 8 of 38 in the spring and summer, $P<.001$).

Young children with a strong HLA-DQ–defined genetic risk of T1DM show signs of beta-cell autoimmunity more often than those with moderate genetic risk. IAA emerged as the first detectable antibody more commonly than any other antibody:

- Insulin may be the primary antigen in most cases of T1DM associated with DR4-DQB1*0302 haplotype
- Seasonal variation in beta-cell autoimmunity suggests that infection may participate in induction of such autoimmunity.

Nielsen JH, Haase TN, Jaksch C, et al. Impact of fetal and neonatal environment on beta cell function and development of diabetes. Acta Obstet Gynecol Scand 2014;93:1109–22.

Global epidemic of diabetes

- Health threat
- High health care expenses.

Dramatic increase in incidence of T1DM must involve environmental factors.

Concept of the thrifty phenotype

- Intrauterine environment during pregnancy affects gene expression
- Persists until adulthood
- Causes metabolic diseases such as obesity and type 2 diabetes mellitus.

Normal pregnancy influences beta cells in both the mother and the fetus.

Diabetes, obesity, overnutrition, or undernutrition during and after pregnancy may affect adaption to insulin demand later in life.

Nutrients and gut microbiota influence appetite regulation, mitochondrial activity, and the immune system that affects beta cell growth and function. The possible role of epigenetic changes in transgenerational transmission of adverse programming is a threatening aspect with regard to the global diabetes epidemic.

Uusitalo U, Liu X, Yang J, et al. Association of early exposure of probiotics and islet autoimmunity in the TEDDY study. JAMA Pediatr 2016;170:20–8.

Probiotics support healthy gut microbiota, affecting immunologic responses to environmental exposures. The hypothesis is that probiotics could be used to prevent development of T1DM-associated islet autoimmunity.

Study: Ongoing prospective cohort of probiotic use during year 1 of life and islet cell autoimmunity among children identified to be at increased genetic risk of T1DM

- Started September 1, 2004
- 6 clinical centers (1 each in Colorado, Georgia-Florida, and Washington; 1 each in Finland, Germany, and Sweden)
- Subjects were followed up for T1DM-related autoantibodies.
- Blood samples were collected (every 3 months for age 3–48 months, then every 6 months) to identify persistent islet autoimmunity (monitoring)

- Infant feeding
- Probiotic supplementation

Association between probiotic use and islet autoimmunity

- Assessed by country
- Adjusting for family history of T1DM
- HLA-DR-DQ genotypes
- Sex
- Birth order
- Mode of delivery
- Exclusive breastfeeding
- Birth year
- Child's antibiotic use
- Diarrheal history
- Maternal age
- Probiotic use
- Smoking.

Altogether, 8676 infants with an eligible genotype were enrolled in the follow-up study before the age of 4 months.

The final sample included 7473 children with the age range of 4 to 10 years (as of October 31, 2014).

Results: Early probiotic supplementation (at the age of 0–27 days) was associated with decreased risk of islet autoimmunity, compared with probiotic supplementation after 27 days, or with no probiotic supplementation (hazard ratio [HR] 0.66, 95% CI 0.46–0.94). The association was accounted for by children with the DR3/4 genotype (HR 0.40, 95% CI 0.21–0.74) and was absent among other genotypes (HR 0.97, 95% CI 0.62–1.54).

Conclusion: Early probiotic supplementation may reduce risk of islet autoimmunity in children who have highest genetic risk of T1DM.

APPENDIX C. INHERITED CALCIUM DISORDERS—RECENT PUBLICATIONS
Outline by Susan R. Rose, MD

Usardi A, Mamoune A, Nattes E, et al. Progressive development of PTH resistance in patients with inactivating mutations on the maternal allele of GNAS. J Clin Endocrinol Metab 2017;102:1844–50.

Objective: Parathyroid hormone (PTH) resistance was assessed in 20 subjects with iPPSD2 (PHP1A) who were identified because of family history, ectopic ossification, or short stature, and carried a GNAS mutation (retrospective study).

PTH resistance factors include hypocalcemia, hyperphosphatemia, and elevated PTH in the absence of vitamin D deficiency.

Pseudohypoparathyroidism type 1A (PHP1A, or inactivating parathormone [PTH]/PTHrp signaling disorder 2) is caused by mutations in maternal GNAS allele:

- Diagnosis at mean age of 3.9 years
- Mean follow-up of 2 years
- Thyroid-stimulating hormone resistance present at diagnosis of PHP1A in all subjects (13.3 ± 9.0 mIU/L).

Over time, PTH levels increased (179–306 pg/mL, $P<.05$) and calcium levels decreased (2.31–2.21 mmol/L, $P<.05$), with no change in phosphate levels.

Conclusion: In patients with iPPSD2 (PHP1A), PTH resistance and hypocalcemia develop over time.

This points out importance of screening for maternal GNAS mutations when ectopic ossifications are present or there is family history.

Gattineni J. Inherited disorders of calcium and phosphate metabolism. Curr Opin Pediatr 2014;26:215–22.

Inherited disorders of calcium and phosphate homeostasis cause significant morbidity.

Calcium and phosphate homeostasis is tightly regulated in a narrow range due to a vital role in many biological processes.

Identification of calcium-sensing receptor (CaSR) mutations has improved understanding of hypocalcemic and hypercalcemic conditions.

Mutations of Fgf23, Klotho, and phosphate transporter genes cause disorders of phosphate metabolism.

Insights into mode of inheritance and pathophysiology will aid in early diagnosis and early institution of therapy.

Ramasamy I. Inherited disorders of calcium homeostasis. Clin Chim Acta 2008;394:22–41.

A complicated homeostatic mechanism (including PTH and vitamin D) maintains consistent extracellular calcium ion levels:
- Recent concerns about vitamin D deficiency as a global health issue
- Causes of rickets include dietary calcium deficiency and inherited disorders of vitamin D and phosphorus metabolism.
- Vitamin D-resistant syndromes
  ○ Hereditary defects in metabolic activation of vitamin D
  ○ Mutations in the vitamin D receptor.

Vitamin D receptor regulates gene expression through zinc finger–mediated DNA binding and protein–protein interaction.

CaSR is key in calcium homeostasis:
- Loss of function mutations in CaSR
  ○ Heterozygous: familial benign hypocalciuric hypercalcemia
  ○ Homozygous: neonatal severe hyperparathyroidism
- Gain of function mutations in CaSR cause the opposite effect
  ○ Autosomal dominant hypocalcemia.

Mouse models using targeted gene disruption strategies have been valuable in studying the effect of CaSR mutations in the vitamin D activation pathway.

New treatment approaches
- Allosteric modulators of CaSR
- Vitamin D analogues inducing unusual structural conformations on the vitamin D receptor.

Ward BK, Magno AL, Walsh JP, et al. The role of the calcium-sensing receptor in human disease. Clin Biochem 2012;45:943–53.

The CaSR was described in 1993.

CaSR has a pivotal role familial hypocalciuric hypercalcemia (FHH):
- Ability to activate different signaling pathways in a ligand-specific and tissue-specific manner.

CaSR plays diverse and crucial roles both in calcium homeostasis and in tissues and biological processes unrelated to calcium balance:

- Disorders of calcium homeostasis (FHH, neonatal severe hyperparathyroidism, autosomal dominant hypocalcemia, primary and secondary hyperparathyroidism, hypercalcemia of malignancy)
- Breast and colorectal cancer (CaSR seems to play a tumor suppressor role), Alzheimer's disease, pancreatitis, diabetes mellitus, hypertension, and bone and gastrointestinal disorders.

CaSR agonists or antagonists (calcimimetics and calcilytics) and other drugs mediated through the CaSR have potential therapeutic utility in hyperparathyroidism, osteoporosis, and gastrointestinal disease.

Stokes VJ, Nielsen MF, Hannan FM, et al. Hypercalcemic disorders in children. J Bone Miner Res 2017. https://doi.org/10.1002/jbmr.3296.

Hypercalcemia is serum calcium concentration greater than 2 standard deviations greater than normal mean.

Presentation of hypercalcemic disorders

- Hypotonia
- Poor feeding
- Vomiting
- Constipation
- Abdominal pain
- Lethargy
- Polyuria
- Dehydration
- Failure to thrive
- Seizures
- Renal failure
- Pancreatitis
- Reduced consciousness
- Psychiatric symptoms.

Causes of hypercalcemia in children

- PTH-dependent or PTH-independent
- Congenital or acquired.

PTH-independent hypercalcemia (suppressed PTH)

- More common in children than PTH-dependent hypercalcemia
- Acquired causes of PTH-independent hypercalcemia
- Hypervitaminosis, granulomatous disorders, and endocrinopathies
- Congenital syndromes
- Idiopathic infantile hypercalcemia, Williams syndrome, and inborn errors of metabolism.

PTH-dependent hypercalcemia

- Usually caused by parathyroid tumors or primary hyperparathyroidism
  - Isolated nonsyndromic and nonhereditary
  - Hereditary hypercalcemic disorder, such as FHH, neonatal severe primary hyperparathyroidism, familial isolated primary hyperparathyroidism, and multiple endocrine neoplasia
- Tertiary hyperparathyroidism from renal failure or in treatment of hypophosphatemic rickets.

Acquired causes of PTH-dependent hypercalcemia in neonates

- Maternal hypocalcemia
- Extracorporeal membrane oxygenation.

Advances in identifying genetic causes are adding to understanding of underlying biological pathways and improved diagnosis.

Management of symptomatic hypercalcemia includes fluids, antiresorptive medications, and parathyroid surgery.

Printed and bound by CPI Group (UK) Ltd, Croydon, CR0 4YY

03/10/2024

01040495-0013